Guinea Pig Doctors

GUINEA PIG DOCTORS

THE DRAMA OF MEDICAL RESEARCH THROUGH SELF-EXPERIMENTATION

Jon Franklin and
John Sutherland, M.D.

WILLIAM MORROW AND COMPANY, INC.

NEW YORK   1984

Copyright © 1984 by Jon Franklin and John Sutherland, M.D.

All rights reserved. No part of this book may be reproduced or utilized in any form or by any means, electronic or mechanical, including photocopying, recording or by any information storage and retrieval system, without permission in writing from the Publisher. Inquiries should be addressed to William Morrow and Company, Inc., 105 Madison Avenue, New York, N.Y. 10016.

Library of Congress Cataloging in Publication Data

Franklin, Jon.
  Guinea pig doctors.

  Includes index.
  1. Self-experimentation in medicine.   2. Physicians—
Biography.   I. Sutherland, John.   II. Title.   [DNLM:
1. Physicians—Biography.   2. Research personnel—
Biography.   3. Research—History.   4. History of
medicine, Modern.   WZ 112 F832g]
R853.S44F73   1984   619'.98   83-19477
ISBN 0-688-02666-4

Printed in the United States of America

First Edition

1 2 3 4 5 6 7 8 9 10

BOOK DESIGN BY ELLEN LO GIUDICE

TO LUCILLE SUTHERLAND,
for love and encouragement

ACKNOWLEDGMENTS

The authors owe a debt of gratitude to many people who, over the years, aided and abetted them in their fascination with and labors over *Guinea Pig Doctors*.

The original inspiration stemmed from the selfless autoexperiment performed by Dr. William Harrington at Barnes Hospital in St. Louis. Dr. Harrington's actions caught the imagination of Dr. John Sutherland, who, at the time, was an even younger physician-scientist at Barnes.

Dr. Sutherland nourished the inspiration over the better part of a lifetime before beginning to seriously develop his research into the guinea pig doctors in the late 1970s. He was encouraged to write the book by his clinical chief, Dr. Peter Wiernik, who was then the director of the National Cancer Institute's clinical research arm at University Hospital in Baltimore.

It was Dr. Wiernik who, having worked with reporter Jon Franklin of *The Evening Sun* on a number of medical stories, introduced the co-authors. From that introduction stemmed a long, fruitful, and mutually educational association culminating in the completion of this manuscript.

In the course of the research, the authors benefited greatly from the knowledge and wisdom of a number of health science researchers who were familiar with one aspect of the stories or another.

Among those to whom the authors are particularly indebted are Dr. José Whittembury, of the University of Peru Cayetano Heredia, and Dr. José Ordóñez, of the University of Maryland Cancer Center. Without their help, the story of Daniel Carrión would not have emerged as the powerful tale it is.

Likewise, Professor Dr. Hermann Eyer, of the Max von Pettenkofer Institute in Munich, provided invaluable assistance in the preparation of the Pettenkofer story. We are also grateful for the help of Dr. Ruth Purtilo, of the University of Nebraska.

Dr. Juan del Regato, of University of Florida, was instrumental in the composition of the Jesse Lazear story.

A similar debt of gratitude is owed to Miss Virginia Minnich, of Barnes Hospital in St. Louis, and Dr. William Hollingsworth, of the San Diego Veterans Administration Hospital. They were responsible for the addition of valuable details and perspective that Dr. Harrington, in modesty, declined to supply.

A number of others were equally invaluable in providing editorial advice, encouragement, and friendly shoulders to cry on. They include Alan Doelp, Jo Bruen, Lynn Scheidhauer, Cathy Franklin, Dianne Tomelden, and the ever-present ghost of G. Vern Blasdell.

We wrote and rewrote the manuscript on a very excellent Compucorp word processor, an experience that makes us wonder how we ever got by with mere typewriters. We are grateful to Bob Bogar, Chuck Cavolo and Mark Zutkoff for all their good advice and cybernetic hand holding.

Finally, we are especially appreciative of the acumen of our fine editor at William Morrow and Company, Laurie Lister, her equally professional associate, Deborah Baker, and our copy editor, Bruce M. Giffords.

Though the above-named individuals share credit for all that is good about this book, they cannot in fairness be blamed for its failings. Those, as always, are the sole responsibility of the authors.

JON FRANKLIN
JOHN SUTHERLAND, M.D.

Baltimore, 1983

CONTENTS

Introduction

In the late 1970s medical scientists at the Stehlin Research Foundation in Houston, Texas, discovered that large doses of a natural substance called thymidine could dramatically shrink cancers in mice.

The news was a bombshell in the cancer research community, not only because thymidine got startling results but also because it wasn't the usual, highly poisonous antitumor agent. Quite the opposite—thymidine was known to be essential, although at low levels, to human life. It was, in fact, present in every living cell.

It was an exceptional drug, and it posed some head-scratching questions to the bureaucrats in faraway Washington.

Federal regulations had been written with the usual, toxic anticancer drug in mind, and they stipulated that all new agents had to be extensively tested for their safety before they could be given to humans.

The safety testing typically consumed perhaps two years of work, and only when that work was completed could the drug be tried on humans. Unfortunately, by that time many of the patients whom the regulations had been written to protect had already died of their tumors.

Thymidine, an old and well-studied substance with no known or theoretical side effects, threw this deadly irony into sharp focus. Dr. Beppino Giovanella, the senior scientist on the thymidine project in Houston, argued passionately that the usual rules should be suspended in this instance.

He reminded his superiors in Washington again and again that the drug in question was *an apparently harmless chemical that seemed to be curing cancer in mice!* And he reminded them that cancer patients were dying every day, at the rate of about one a minute.

Sure, thymidine probably wouldn't work in people. How many things were ever as good as they looked at first? But if there was no reason not to, why not skip the safety tests and find out quickly? If it didn't work, at least they wouldn't raise everyone's hopes and squander several million dollars of precious cancer research money. And if it did work . . .

If it did work!

Consider how many lives might be saved if the Food and Drug Administration was bold now! Think how many lives would be lost if it hesitated and stood on the letter of the law! *Imagine how many patients would die needlessly while the drug that might have saved them was given, instead, to mice, rats, guinea pigs, dogs, and finally monkeys?*

It was a powerful argument, and Beppino Giovanella was a persuasive man. For a brief time, the Food and Drug Administration committee wavered, debating the possibility.

It was true, as Dr. Giovanella said, that thymidine was a natural substance. But it existed in the body only in very small quantities, and it had taken massive doses to shrink tumors in mice. There was no proof that huge amounts were safe for humans. No proof at all.

Exasperated, Dr. Giovanella argued that even so, the risk seemed slight. After all, the first patients would be terminal cases, wouldn't they? The chance that they would die of their cancer was 100 percent, wasn't it? Why not explain the risk to the patients, then, and let *them* decide?

The FDA officials debated a little longer, but they found that the letter of the law was quite clear, while the spirit was opaque. New drugs simply couldn't be tried in humans until safety trials had been completed and the proper forms had been filled out and filed in all the specified places. Nowhere in law, regulation, or precedent was there an exception, and what if someone died? What would happen then? Bureaucratic heads would roll, that was what would happen.

So the answer had to be no.

But, Dr. Giovanella argued . . .

Sorry, the board said. The answer was no, and that was final.

. . . but weren't there times, Dr. Giovanella went on anyway . . . weren't there times when a scientist, even a modern scientist-bureaucrat, was called on to exercise judgment for the betterment of the human race? Consider the big potential payoff. . . .

No, said the board. No, no, and no.

And so, as Dr. Giovanella sat in his office in Texas, fuming at the *t*-crossing and *i*-dotting timidity of bureaucracies, the bureaucrats themselves began moving forward with all deliberate speed, planning the call for proposals that would be written, drawing up lists of scientists who would have to review and debate the interim and final results, and otherwise making preparations to fulfill the law of the land.

Then safety testing would begin, perhaps, on mice and rats. In the fullness of time the scientists would move on to dogs and, again, committees would meet. Reports would be submitted and analyzed. Lawyers and statisticians would be consulted. Budgets would be considered, reconsidered, submitted, rewritten, compromised, finalized, and filed. New experiments would be planned, this time on primates.

But in Houston, Dr. Giovanella's fury had given way to cold calculation.

Okay, he reasoned. The folks in Washington were in the catbird seat. They could refuse to authorize the immediate use of thymidine on patients if they wanted, and their decision would be respected throughout the scientific world.

But there was at least one human being over which Washington, in its silliness, didn't have complete control—and that was Beppino Giovanella. Beppino Giovanella could commit suicide if he liked. He could throw himself from a bridge, blow his brains out . . . drown himself, if it pleased him, in thymidine.

In fact, he said, laughing off the alarmed protests of his co-workers, there was no danger. He wrote up his own experimental protocol, arranged for the proper tests, collected the necessary witnesses, filled a beaker with thymidine, held it up to the light, silently toasted the muse of science and rationality, and drank.

Nothing happened, of course, so the next day he drank a larger dose. The following day he drank more, and the day after that he drank still more. As the experiment proceeded, he collected carefully labeled samples of his blood and urine, to be forwarded to the skeptics in Washington.

Each day he drank more and more until, finally, he got a reaction: cramps and diarrhea. Surprised, he dashed for a bathroom.

That, he had to admit when the attack was over, was a problem.

Not that a cancer patient would complain of a few abdominal miseries, and loose bowels were certainly preferable to death . . . but the diarrhea was washing the thymidine out of his system. Dr. Giovanella wanted to push the experiment further, to drive his blood levels of thymidine up so high that his point would be made all the way to Washington. The problem was that his intestines refused to absorb enough.

He would have to try the most logical alternative. He would inject the stuff directly into his veins.

Not that intravenous administration was much of a problem. It was, in fact, no problem at all. It was easy to rig an IV and to let the thymidine trickle directly into his circulatory system. The doses got larger and larger and larger, and the blood levels went ever higher.

By the time he was satisfied that he had made his point, his body was almost saturated with thymidine. He had consumed so much that tiny, needlelike crystals suddenly appeared in the bottle containing his final urine sample. They were composed of a thymidine metabolite, crystallizing out of the saturated liquid as it cooled.

A few days later a beaming, satisfied, vindicated, and obviously healthy Beppino Giovanella presented the FDA committee members with dramatic evidence that thymidine, whether or not it cured cancer, posed no danger to the patient.

Now . . . bureaucracies are faceless things, ponderous paper mills that grind slowly, disembodied creatures without the capacity to blush. So it cannot be said that the FDA was embarrassed. But it can be said that it stopped dead in its tracks.

Thanks to the moxie of a Texas researcher, the government halted the safety-testing process, briefly pondered the obvious, and reversed itself. In a matter of days, thymidine was trickling into the veins of dying cancer patients at several research institutions across the country.

It is a matter of historical record, of course, that thymidine didn't cure cancer. The results of the first clinical trials were disappointing. Apparently, the substance has only a modest effect in humans. So the clinical trials proved no more than a footnote in the history of cancer research, indicating that, as it's said, "more research is needed." It also stands as one more testimony to the difficulties inherent in trying to cure human cancer by means of experiments on rats and mice.

Though Dr. Giovanella had hoped the drug would be more useful, he was philosophical about the outcome. That, he explained to reporters, was the way it was in science. Besides, a negative outcome didn't make his self-experiment a failure.

In the narrow world of cancer research, Beppino Giovanella's experiment on himself accomplished two things. First, he saved a reluctant government perhaps a million dollars or more—a substantial sum when applied to other experiments. Second, and more important, he saved time . . . the wasted time of safety-testing a chemical that would never be used anyway. And time, of course, is the one thing cancer patients don't have.

In a broader sense, there was a third and more general benefit as well. The drama that took place in Houston was widely reported, and it demonstrated a truth about medical science that the public is all too often inclined to forget.

In a society that emphasizes procedure over people, it is popular to visualize medical science as a logical process, as an accumulation of data and knowledge that proceeds in the direction of truth without regard to the egos, personalities, hunches, and convictions of the human beings who do the experiments.

But science is no such abstraction. It is only superficially delineated by regulation, and it isn't, in the end, ruled by committee. It is instead a human enterprise, a quiet workaday war against ignorance that spends most of its time bogged down in confusion and procedure . . . and then surges dramatically ahead as a result of individual human vision, faith, and courage. No one illustrates this truth more dramatically than the scientist who wagers his life on the correctness of his theory.

Beppino Giovanella is uncommon only because his auto-experiment became part of the official record and, when the drug was released, appeared in newspapers and television reports. In fact, it is almost routine for medical scientists to try out their ideas first on themselves.

Their reasons for doing so grow out of the age in which they live and work. The modern scientist, frustrated by the elaborate rules of the multilayered science and health bureaucracy, often experiments on himself simply to avoid having to waste time dickering with his human experimentation committee. It is simpler for him to draw his own blood, monitor his own body, and consume his own drugs.

Scientists readily talk about this to one another, and will often confide in a friendly reporter—providing, of course, that it's off the record. After all, they say, it doesn't sound very scientific. . . .

As a result, too few people outside of science are aware of the dramatic and sometimes pivotal role that autoexperimentation has played in the development of modern medicine.

It is a subject that raises awkward questions. What are the ethics, after all, of outfoxing one's own lawfully established human-experimentation committee? What would Occupational Safety and Health Administration say? If the scientist kills himself, should his wife and children receive workmen's compensation? What about social security? Would those who assisted him be open to charges of murder?

Beneath those ethical and legal questions lurks a darker,

more substantive issue of scientific method. How involved can a scientist become in his own experiment, how obsessed by an idea, before he loses the ability to look at the results with the necessary dispassion? Does the scientist who conducts an autoexperiment take a chance on actually obscuring the truth he's trying to uncover?

And why, for that matter, does the idea occur to him in the first place? To what extent was Dr. Giovanella's ego, and his conviction that he was smarter than the committee that overruled him, a determining factor in his decision? He told reporters that ego didn't enter into his decision at all—but then, was he the most appropriate judge?

Such enigmas aside, the issue itself isn't in doubt. The scientist's own body is . . . well . . . handy.

He controls it. He can keep what he does with it a secret. When he experiments on himself, no citizen can call him inhumane. And, if challenged later, he can point to a long list of researchers in whose footsteps he follows.

Since the dawn of modern medicine in the 1700s, the tradition of autoexperimentation has been part of the mainstream of scientific history. Then as now, explorations on the frontier were guided by guess and clouded by ignorance, and if at times the stories you are about to read touch on the bizarre . . . who can say that the science of our own time will fare better in the enlightened perspective of the 21st century?

At the time, at least, the autoexperimenters of the past thought their theories, actions, and conclusions were a logical extension of the science of their day. Like all other human beings they were creatures of their times.

As a result, their self-experiments gave us more than mere facts, proofs, and theories. The guinea pig doctors bequeathed us their stories as well—lenses through which we can watch the birth, childhood, and adolescence of the most glorious and at the same time most fallible of all sciences.

What century but the 18th, for instance, could produce a grave robber who kept a pet bull to wrestle with—and who ushered anatomy into the modern world?

John Hunter was a giant of his time, but his time was an age of the darkest ignorance. It was somehow natural that he should push his impatient intellect far beyond the limits of its resolution, and that he would accidentally prove a theorem far older than science . . . a theorem about curiosity, and cats.

And there was Daniel Carrión, of all the guinea pig doctors the one most obviously driven by history. Mesmerized by an outmoded Spanish chivalry, caught up in the patriotic fervor of the young men around him, he guessed the deadly secret of the canyon—and paid for it with his life.

Then there was Horace Wells, who could soothe everyone's pain but his own, and Jesse Lazear, who wanted desperately to succeed whatever the price.

But of all the guinea pig doctors it was Herr Professor Doctor Max von Pettenkofer, the failed actor, who explained it most dramatically.

"If I die in the service of science," he said, holding the flask high for all to see, "my death will be, like that of a soldier, on the field of honor."

The sentiment, however well spoken, would have echoed more loudly in history had the liquid he drank not contained deadly cholera bacteria. Throughout, the history of autoexperimentation is laced with those same nagging questions posed again by the modern ethicists. And always, in each story, the tradition reflects the contradictions of history.

It took a Werner Forssmann, a product of the same culture as Adolf Hitler, to boldly contemplate pushing a catheter into his own heart. But he lacked the more subtle courage to turn his back on the Führer.

With each turn of history, science changes and, along

with it, so does the practice of autoexperimentation.

As we approach the present we enter the time in which scientist-doctors first begin to glimpse the incredible, hitherto unsuspected complexity of biology. It is against this backdrop that young Bill Harrington, a student in St. Louis, finds himself locked in mortal struggle against the dimly guessed, deadly intricacies of the human immune system.

And through it all, the nagging questions arise again and again. Is the scientist who drinks a flask containing cholera germs, or who inoculates himself with mysterious antigens . . . is such a scientist, wedded to his own ideas, the best judge of their risk?

The stories of the guinea pig doctors remind us that scientists, too, are subject to blind faith . . . and that theories, in science, are the civilian equivalent of mother, country, and kin. A powerful idea can mesmerize a doctor into overlooking his own mortality.

Further, the guinea pig doctors haven't always had a benign effect. John Hunter's dead hand stifled research on venereal disease for decades—why look for the answer, if it's already known? And Herr Professor Doktor Max von Pettenkofer's error kept the bacterial theory of disease from being fully accepted until well into the 20th century.

But for all that, the stories of the guinea pig doctors trace a golden thread through the fabric of science. There is ego there—ego aplenty. There is ignorance, there is miscalculation, there is bias . . . but nowhere in any of the stories will you find cowardice in the face of an idea. Herr Professor Doktor Max von Pettenkofer may have been a pompous fool, and as a soldier in the service of science he may have been a casualty, but no one can say he shrank from the battle.

Even today, Beppino Giovanella's defiant voice, speaking the language of action, rises above the murmur of ethical debate. It was, after all, his life. He could do with it what he pleased, and if he was wrong it was only he who would pay.

In the end the guinea pig doctors who guess wrong do pay, often with their lives. But success is a different matter.

Bill Harrington, haunted for years by the specter of a dead girl on a mortuary slab, succeeded in discovering the nature of her disease. Tens of thousands of victims of idiopathic thrombocytopenic purpura will live longer, healthier lives as a result. Horace Wells, regardless of the personal tragedy he endured, left us the priceless gift of anesthesia.

Jesse Lazear's experiment, as stupidly risky as it might have been, provided the key to the control of yellow fever—thereby saving uncounted lives and making it possible to build the Panama Canal.

Finally, in the age of roaring machines, Dr. John Paul Stapp strapped himself into a rocket sled, streaked off across the desert at close to the speed of sound, and slammed into the equivalent of a brick wall. The impact was almost great enough to tear the retinas from his eyes, but the results drove home a point that too few are willing, even now, to hear: *Seat belts save lives.*

So while politicians and ethicists will debate the merits of autoexperimentation, scientists as varied as John Hunter and Beppino Giovanella will continue to look inward for their judgments, and to view their own bodies as a court of last resort.

It's my life, Beppino Giovanella said. *I can do whatever I want with it.*

The rest of us can reflect on their stories and conclude that when a guinea pig doctor fails, the tragedy that results is essentially a private matter.

But when he succeeds, the benefits accrue to us all.

HOW THE GHOULS GOT
JOHN HUNTER'S HEART

The body-snatchers they have come
And made a snatch at me;
It's very hard them kind of men
Won't let a body be.

—TOM HOOD

After they were certain he was dead, the ghouls wrapped the body in a blanket and put it in a sedan chair. Porters lifted the chair and carried it out of the building and down the steps to the street. Matthew Baillie, the dead man's nephew, and Everard Home, who was a chief ghoul, walked behind. Several lesser ghouls and apprentices followed at a respectful distance.

The now dead man had arrived in a coach, and as the sedan chair with his remains reached the street the coachman clicked his tongue at the horses and the empty vehicle moved in behind the apprentices.

The streets of London were bustling with carts and carriages. Mongrel dogs ran between the clattering, iron-rimmed wheels of the vehicles, pausing to sniff curiously at the piles of garbage and excrement in the gutters. A sharp, cold edge in the air hinted at the coming winter.

The traffic parted for the procession of death as it moved east, toward Piccadilly Circus. As it passed the up-

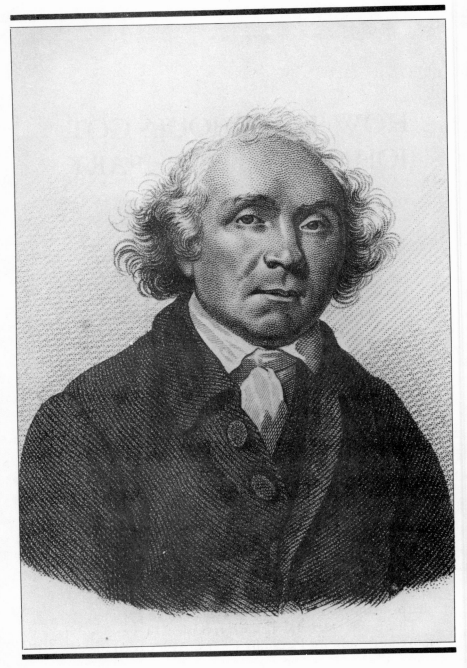

DR. JOHN HUNTER

per-class row houses across from Hyde Park, young servant girls called the children to them.

The ghouls, they whispered. *Here come the ghouls.*

The children clung to the protective skirts, eyes wide,
watching the sedan chair and the stony-faced men who
followed it.

The news traveled ahead. By the time the ghouls
reached Leicester Square, it was uncharacteristically
empty. Curtains moved in the windows of the houses and
hidden eyes watched. The chair stopped in front of a
building at the middle of the block.

The curtains fluttered.

*It's Dr. Hunter. Dr. Hunter is dead, and look at who followed
the body. He was one of them, but they want his heart anyway,
to put in a jar, just like he said they would.*

For a moment the procession stood idly in the street, in
front of the house, and then the front door opened. William Clift, Dr. Hunter's chief assistant, appeared briefly in
the doorway, his face white and stricken. He stepped
aside as the porters brought the sedan chair up the steps
and into the house. The carriage moved on down the
street, the horses' hooves clip-clopping hollowly on the
cobblestones, heading for the stables.

As soon as the body and its entourage were inside the
house, Dr. Hunter's young assistant closed the door and
shot the bolt. As the porters stood for a moment in the
hallway, he stepped to the sedan chair and lifted the
blanket from the dead man's face. He met the sightless
eyes for a moment and then, tears streaming down his
face, he turned away.

The sedan chair lurched forward and the ghouls followed it, grimly, through the house. Their faces were set
and blank. He had been one of them, and their duty was
clear.

It was by his own hand, by the force of his own will,
that it had come to this.

It was true that, born one year after Isaac Newton died, John Hunter arrived in the world in what historians might describe as the modern age. New ideas were abroad in London and Paris, and the world was changing.

But the impact of the new age wasn't yet felt outside the universities. England's witchcraft statutes were still in effect, alchemy retained its influence, astrologers were more honored than physicians, and Charles Darwin would not be born for another century. The sweet, logical song of modern science wasn't yet heard in the Scottish farming village of Kilbride, near the city of Glasgow. The Middle Ages still lay across the farmers' pious minds like an obscuring fog.

They recognized, almost from the beginning, that John Hunter was somehow different. They would never have guessed that his heart would end up in a ghoul's bottle, but even as a toddler he was clearly, well . . . The Hunters were a fine old family, and John's father was a gentleman, and you were careful what you said about a gentleman's son, even a dullard third son . . . but still . . . a dullard was what he was, without doubt. Vacant, preoccupied, addled, and certain, virtually certain, to grow up worthless.

They were, in a sense, correct. As a young child John was ignorant even of the judgment that had been passed on him. But his apparent lack of interest was just that: apparent. If his mind failed to grasp the affairs of those around him, it was because those affairs were obviously petty and boring. John's handicap was that in this waning of the Great Medieval Night his brain perceived the morning light, and was blinded by it.

It was easy, in a time so innocent of truth, to be fascinated by the existence of questions, of endless questions, of the song of curiosity that wafted through his brain and beckoned, irresistibly . . . from the barnyard.

Chickens were different from pigs, in some ways, he noted.

Chickens had feathers and pigs had coarse hair.

Both had legs, but chickens had only two—unless you counted the wings, which were sort of . . . legs for the air. Of course, chickens couldn't fly very far. They were much like pigs in that respect.

The siren sang from the waters of the pond, and she flirted with him through the eyes of a lazy carp. Her melodies whipped through the pasture on the wind and called to him from the throats of soaring hawks. Through curiosity and imagination the child followed her, not as a poet but as a scientist.

When the hawks had finished with a rabbit, and when the insects had cleaned the bones, you could see the way the skeleton was articulated. There were rubbery cushions where the joints rubbed together.

Curious. The bones of a rabbit's foot were much different from those of a chicken's, though both creatures could move very fast.

The siren called from the earth, where tiny ants dug in the soil, and from the fragile sprouts of springtime grass. She sang to him through the mouths of birds, whispered from the brook, sighed in the trees.

She did not, however, call from the schoolhouse.

Books?

What were books?

Books were dead plants, with the shape pounded out of them, glued together with the hooves of worn-out horses, stained with cryptic symbols. There was more to be seen in a robin's egg than in books . . . and more, far, far more, in a live trout on the end of a taut line, twisting and dodging in the current, sizzling over a fire.

If you needed to know a truth deeper than the taste of fresh trout, you didn't go to books. You went to a carpenter or a blacksmith, and sat, and asked questions.

Go to school, his parents demanded.

He was a source of embarrassment to his elder brother, William, who had always been a good student. William pleaded with John. Did he want to grow up to be a rogue?

His father, in desperation, pursued the problem to a more rudimentary part of the anatomy. John screamed in pain and fear and yes, beatings could make him go to school, for a while. But beatings couldn't make dead books come alive, and couldn't make subtraction suddenly metamorphose, like a caterpillar, into something fine and interesting.

Eventually, even his own family resigned themselves to the judgment of the community. It was easier to simply accept that John was dim-witted, a little.

At least, they could tell themselves, big brother William was different. He was a serious student, studying in London, a credit to his father, but John was . . . in the eyes of the community, John was a pity.

The young man could fix a wagon or fork hay, it was true, but in honesty he wasn't one of the finer sorts. You wouldn't see John Hunter in church, for instance, and he drank. He drank and brawled. He was the kind of lad you wouldn't be surprised to see lying in a muddy gutter. . . . He would make a poor son-in-law.

It was not inconsistent with that judgment that John Hunter's final house, the scene of his happiest work, would be equipped with heavy shutters that bolted from the inside. The shutters protected him and his family from the angry mobs that sometimes gathered, with rope and torches, to scream for his blood.

But the day the ghouls brought his body home, no servant rushed to close those shutters.

The siren had given him no peace and he, in his atheistic weakness, had never undertaken a moral struggle against her. So she had toyed with him, taunted him, driven him, turned him into a ghoul, and, in the end, she had killed him. This day the shutters needn't be bolted because the mob would raise no hand in protest. It was only appropriate now that she should have his heart in a jar.

The judgment of the Scottish farmers was a powerful thing, and while John could ignore it as a child, as a young man he found it a burden. Had he been a true dullard he could have accepted it but, since his ignorance was only apparent, the requirements of society finally began to force their way into his protesting mind. By the time he reached twenty, he could no longer ignore his own future.

Would he simply live out his life, follow the path set for him, grow old, and die a drunkard's warm death in a snowbank? No. As adrenaline and testosterone flowed in the young man's blood, the imperative of manhood took hold. No. He cared nothing for the judgment of the farmers, but he wouldn't live a dullard's life. Somehow, in some way, he would make a mark.

But not there, not in the village.

He and his questions weren't welcome in the village. He would flee, as bright, misunderstood young men in his time and place often did, to London.

It was 1748, and from London, George II ruled all that was touched by the sea. His shipping fleets sailed for Africa with trade goods, from there to the West Indies with slaves, to North America with rum, and back to England with cotton, tobacco, and raw materials. The merchant ships, and the men-of-war that protected them, had bound the world with the chains of commerce.

London was the center of the universe, and its streets were lit by the light of the new age. In London they spoke of scientifically breeding cattle and sheep. In London they talked of the Frenchman Voltaire. In London, Blackstone was a judge, Chippendale a furniture maker. In London, Samuel Johnson wrote that curiosity was one of the permanent and certain characteristics of the human mind.

Equally important, John's elder brother William was now a teacher of anatomy in London. William, who had never quite given up on John, was quick to offer him a job. It wasn't a good job, he explained apologetically, but . . .

John accepted. In London, somehow, he would find his destiny.

John's visions of London were accurate, as far as they went. The empire was in full flower, but Samuel Johnson's society had a soft, putrescent underbelly. It stank of gin.

As a Scotsman, John was familiar with the power of distilled spirits. He himself drank to what the gentlemen farmers considered excess, and even his mother took a tot in the morning, for her health. But nothing had prepared him for the gin mills of London.

The gin mania had begun about the time of John's birth, when the crown decided that, as a subsidy to England's grain farmers, gin shouldn't be taxed. Because beer and wine were heavily taxed, the population quickly switched to the stronger, and more addictive, gin.

The men who successfully ruled the empire hadn't fathomed the hopelessness of their own poor, and hadn't anticipated the succor that they would find in gin. By the time they understood what had happened and reimposed the tax, it was too late. Alcoholism had already taken hold.

John was horrified by the drunkenness that was visible, it seemed, everywhere. Everywhere there were dirty little dens that advertised, "Drunk for a penny, dead drunk for two pence, clean straw twice a week." Half-dressed women lay slumped in doorways, beggars staggered at every street corner, and able-bodied men squandered their days slumped across barroom tables, while intoxicated mothers weaned their funny-looking offspring on gin.

The problem, by the time John arrived, went far beyond mere drunkenness. There was violence everywhere, and the funny-looking babies, having grown to adulthood, were taunted by drunken crowds as they were led to the gallows. And, as if to underscore the immorality of the conditions, the pox was widespread.

The pox was sexually transmitted so it made sense, in London, that it would become known as the French disease, morbus Gallicus. The French in turn called it the Italian disease, and the Italians blamed it on the Indians of the New World . . . a disease in return, perhaps, for the deadly measles that the Europeans carried to America.

The Europeans were as sensitive to the pox as the Indians were to measles, and many died of its fevers. Though resistance was already beginning to build by the time John Hunter was born, it was still an occasional killer.

It didn't kill you now, the wisdom went, but sometimes it might as well. The pox, if you were unlucky, could rot the organ of manhood. Such rumors were a strong inducement to adolescent chastity.

Some said the pox was one disease, and others said it was really two similar diseases. At twenty, John had no opinion either way. His strong ambition, concerning the pox, was to escape it.

Not that his employment in his brother's anatomy school allowed him much leisure time to commit the act necessary to catch the pox, nor did the nature of his profession attract ardent women. It was nothing like being a sea captain, or a lieutenant of marines, or even a common seaman.

He could think of himself as an anatomist if he liked, and . . . in technical truth it was no longer criminal to be a ghoul. Of course, it was no longer a capital crime to be a

witch, either, but that didn't stop people from being
witches.

Not that John personally robbed graves. He didn't. He
just answered the alley door.

Sometimes the transaction was conducted openly, in
full view of a half-dozen gawkers. The hangman nervously
stepped inside—but only just inside—to get his money. It
was John's business, not the hangman's, to wrestle the
corpse into the dissecting room and deposit it on a stone
slab.

Whatever it said about the state of society, the fre-
quency of public hangings was a boon to brother William.
The gallows brought him healthy bodies, and they were
by far the best for dissection. The other ones, the ones
that came in the night, were all diseased. But John accepted those, too, since even in those days there weren't
enough healthy bodies to go around to all the would-be
surgeons. John slept right above the dissecting room, so
whenever he heard a rapping in the night he rose from
bed, lit a candle, and answered the door.

Grave robbing was a partnership operation, so there
were usually two men who reeked of gin and poverty, and
they were always in a big hurry to get their burden inside,
and to see the door locked. John inspected the cadaver to
see that it wasn't putrid before paying the men. Everyone
knew that William didn't accept putrid cadavers, but the
kinds of people that robbed graves were rarely the kind of
people you could trust.

When the business had been consummated and the
corpse lay on a stone table, the grave robbers disappeared
into the darkness. After bolting the door, John returned to
the dissecting room to inspect the new specimen. Often it
was dressed in a shroud, but it never had any jewelry on
it. Occasionally the ring finger was missing.

The dissections weren't done in summer, because of the

difficulty of preserving corpses in the heat. So the dissecting room was cold, but even so the air was always laced with the faint, sweet odor of decomposing flesh.

Methodically, John stripped the corpse of its clothes, spread its legs and made an incision in one thigh. He found the main artery and spliced the embalming hose onto it. He also opened a vein so that the blood could drain out. The embalming fluid, a mixture of vermilion and the oils of turpentine, lavender, and rosemary, ran down from an earthenware bowl overhead.

As the fluid displaced the blood John massaged the body vigorously, working the preservative into all the tissues. The chemicals gave the white flesh a faint blush.

The farmers back home wouldn't have been surprised to learn that his ghoulish job didn't disturb John much. He felt no compulsion to either meet or avoid the staring eyes of the cadavers, and his sleep was sound and guiltless. To John, a dead man or woman was no different from a skinned rabbit, a stuck pig, or a hanging side of beef. The farmers would have attributed his indifference to the dullness they thought they saw in his mind, but again they would have been wrong. The thing that protected him, and that allowed him to sleep serenely in the midst of death, was curiosity. It was impossible to be both fascinated and frightened at the same time.

John had come to his brother's dissecting house to work, and work he did. But William knew his brother's unusual weakness, and used it mercilessly to keep his attention.

Look, William said.

Take a leg. That one, there. Make a long incision along the inside of the thigh and peel back the skin and fat. Work down to the fascia, right there . . . the membrane over the muscles. That's the fascia. Split that and lay it back. What you now have before you are the superficial muscles.

Each is attached to a specific place. That big muscle there, the rectus femoris, is attached to the pelvic bone at one end and at the other to the kneecap. See? Now. Detach one end and lay it back. More muscles. Lay them back. See the way the large arteries, veins, and nerves travel deep in the flesh, where they're less likely to be injured? You have to hold the candle steadier than that. There. That's better.

William's knives were sharp, and he taught John to keep them that way. At night John mopped, embalmed, held candles for William, and finally collapsed into bed, exhausted. In the daytime, he stood with the students, four to a cadaver, and listened to William lecture.

As the dissections proceeded, each part was examined minutely. An occasional organ, which had some remarkable and instructive feature, was saved. John would have saved more specimens but for William, who had to approve each one. An anatomy school, he said, was always in danger of turning into a museum, crowded out by jars of fascinating kidneys, hearts, livers, and tongues. William deemed most organs unremarkable, and they were dropped in the bucket that sat, waiting, by the dissection table.

Most of the students came to William's school because they wanted to be apprenticed in surgery, and anatomy school was a necessary precondition to that. For them dismantling a corpse was a means to an end, but for John it was an end in itself.

Nature was full of surprises and puzzles, far too many for a young man to solve. The inside of the belly, for instance, was brightly painted. You slit the belly from the breastbone to the pubis, and made two lateral incisions so you could lay the skin back. Below the skin and a variable amount of fat, you found the muscles of the belly, and noted, as William pointed out from the lectern, that they, like the muscles in the leg, were covered by a membrane, a fascia.

Then you were through the muscles and down to the peritoneum, which lines the abdominal cavity. Beneath that . . . color.

The colon and intestine were light gray, and they sparkled wetly in the light. The small bowel was covered with an apron of bright yellow fat, and there were yellow globules all along the colon. The spleen lay like a dark ruby, in the upper left. The liver was a rich brown.

That was puzzling. Why did nature waste such lavish color on such a dark and private place?

In the name of curiosity, John reduced body after body to buckets of organs and muscles. He consumed the lessons compulsively, and his expertise quickly outstripped that of the other students. The first year in William's anatomy school, John worked and studied. In his second year, he taught.

As he mastered the connections of bone and muscle, John's curiosity naturally moved on to abnormal pathology. Take, for instance, this question of the pox.

As the bodies of murderers, thieves, alcoholics, wastrels, and whores passed beneath John's sharp knife and curious eye, they bore mute testimony to the harshness of life. The ravages of the pox were very apparent. John learned first hand that many of the horror stories he had heard about the pox were true. If you got the pox, your penis might rot. It was rare, but it happened.

Now why, John wondered, did the penis sometimes rot and sometimes not? Why, for that matter, did the symptoms in general vary so widely from victim to victim? Some thought the key was that it wasn't just one disease, but several different ones that all went by the same name.

The enigma of the pox tugged at his mind. Everything he learned about the pox made it seem inconsistent, somehow, with the general theory of disease.

The popular concept of disease had its roots in the dim past, but it had been articulated most clearly by Thomas

Sydenham, an English physician of a century earlier. Sydenham said disease came from "morbid and unwholesome particles" that arose from putrefaction, either within the body or externally, in swamps and low places. The particles were carried in the air, in what he called miasmas.

But the pox was sexually transmitted, apparently, by the direct contact of sexual organs. That meant, in John Hunter's mind, that it wasn't transmitted by miasmas at all. The pox must be caused by a sort of liquid miasma, then . . . a putrid liquid of some kind.

But why, then, were the symptoms so variable—at least in men? In women, you often couldn't tell that the disease was even present.

Sometimes, in some men, the urethra was involved. Then, for several weeks, the victim underwent torture each time he urinated. In another victim, however, the only symptom might be a transitory chancre, or pimple, on the head of the penis. In that case, the victim seemed to have a variety of secondary symptoms after the pimple disappeared. Those symptoms could be treated by rubbing mercury into the thighs.

And then, sometimes, in the odd case, the disease recurred and the penis began to slough away. Mercury didn't seem to help much. A pox-rotted penis was considered remarkable, and wasn't tossed into the waiting pail. With William's permission, it was preserved in a jar.

A ghoul, according to legend, was a creature that robbed graves and consumed the corpse. John's knife laid open body after body. He tore them apart, each in its turn, and his eyes recorded, and his fingers probed, and his mind raced. His curiosity, rather than being satiated, grew apace. Though it was not his purpose, the work moved him inevitably toward the practice of surgery.

It was not, in John's day, a high calling. So closely was it still allied with the barbering trade that German Army surgeons were still required, as part of their duties, to shave their officers. Since there were no anesthetics, surgeons were called to the bedside only when there was no alternative, and they were accompanied by strong men equipped with leather straps to hold the patient down.

With the patient fighting and screaming, surgery in the abdomen was unthinkable, and major operations were confined to the amputation of gangrenous limbs. A surgeon was judged not by delicate fingers but by speed, for if an amputation took more than a few seconds the tormented patient would inevitably die. He often did anyway.

The allied practice of medicine wasn't held in much higher repute, since most serious diseases were effectively untreatable anyway. In Samuel Johnson's London, astrologers and midwives held sway over the popular mind, and even the aristocrats couldn't distinguish between physician and fraud. While physicians and surgeons bickered over who had the better claim to the practice of the healing arts, quackery was rampant. As John Hunter worked in the dissecting house, the queen was being treated by two mountebanks who had abandoned their trades as tinker and tailor in favor of the more lucrative practice of medicine.

But the revolution was coming, and it would turn, as all revolutions must, on passionate characters with inquisitive minds and strong opinions. And as the Scottish farmers had duly noted, John Hunter definitely qualified as passionate.

Though his work in the dissecting house didn't leave him as much free time as he had had at home, London didn't change his personality. When he wasn't buying a felon's body or dismantling the stolen corpse of a matron, he could be found in the beer halls, banging his mug on the table and hurling raucous insults at the performers. And as for opinions . . . ask him about the pox.

The pox?

John Hunter had the pox all figured out.

In his opinion there were two forms. If it began as a pimple on the penis, it took one specific course. The chancre would go away quickly, but two or three weeks later you could expect a sore throat, a skin rash, bone and joint pain, and pox on the skin. Sometimes there'd be a fever as well, and if the fever got high enough, you'd die. If it didn't kill you, though, the pox would finally go away and you'd be cured. You could help the cure along by rubbing mercury into the skin.

The other form was seen when the soft tissue on the interior of the urethra was affected. That was by far the more miserable manifestation of the disease, and if you were unlucky enough to get that form you faced two or three weeks of agony with each urination. Your testicles might get sore. This form, when it affected the female, could cause scarring in the fallopian tubes, and that could cause sterility.

As John would explain to whoever would listen, the existence of two forms misled some people into thinking that the pox was really two diseases, not one. That was wrong, however, dead wrong.

Consider, he explained, that each part of the body was subject to different problems. The skin got warts and boils and various running sores, and was also the home of smallpox and measles. The throat was the seat of hydrophobia and whooping cough, and tuberculosis attacked the lungs. The breasts, the testicles, and the conglomerate glands were the seat of cancer.

So, he continued triumphantly, tissues were different. Obviously, then, and as a fool could see, the different symptoms of the pox arose depending on what tissues were touched by the disease-bearing pus.

If the putrid substance took hold in the firmer tissues on

the outside of the penis, then a firm sore, or chancre, developed, and you had the first form of the disease. If, on the other hand, the putrid substance found its way into the urethra, then the urethra became inflamed and, being a "wet tissue" to start with, produced a liquid discharge.

What could be simpler? A runny disease came from wet, soft tissues; a hard lesion arose from dry, firm tissues. A dunce could see! Mice produced mice, hawks produced fledgling hawks, and swine gave birth only to swine. Like produced like!

What could be more natural, and another round of beer, wench, and let's have more music.

The Scottish farmers at home wouldn't have been surprised to find that John's liking for spirits and song remained strong, and they would have thought his fascination with the pox to be very much in character. But they would have been surprised by the ambition that, in London, began to manifest itself.

By 1753 he had been elected master of anatomy by the surgeon's corporation, but by then he was no longer satisfied by a ghoul's limited existence. The life of a surgeon, by comparison, seemed much broader, and the following year he landed a position as surgeon's assistant at St. George's Hospital. A year later, following his brother's advice that a formal education would make his mind work more clearly, he even enrolled at Oxford.

But in that, William was wrong, and in two months he was back at the anatomy school, wrestling corpses. In the evenings, at the tavern, he explained to his friends that the Oxford professors had tried to make an old woman of him. They wanted him to study Greek and Latin! Imagine! Latin! What could be deader than Latin, out of books?

And yes, another beer.

William allowed John to take back his old job in the anatomy school until he could land another residency, this time at St. George's Hospital. There nobody cared whether he knew Latin or Greek, as long as he kept the charity ward in reasonable order. The appointment left him free to indulge his curiosity without becoming too involved with books.

The trouble with books was, well . . . for instance, some of the books said the pox was a single disease, and others said it was two diseases. You could read that in books, and argue about it, and parrot it back, but you still didn't know anything. If you wanted to understand the pox, or anything else, you had to use your hands, your eyes, and your brain. If you saw patients with the pox, and you thought through the logic of it, then you knew that the pox was a single disease that could affect two tissues. If it affected the dry tissues on the outside of the penis, then it was a dry disease. If it affected the wet tissues of the urethra, then it was a runny disease. The pox was one disease with two manifestations.

In the beginning, it was a student anatomist's guess, but, with time, it became a hypothesis, and with more time the hypothesis became a theory, and the theory became, well . . . in Hunter's view it was plain, obvious fact.

All the world was plain obvious fact, if a man only looked. But he had to look. He couldn't get it out of books. Books were dead plants, with the shape pounded out of them.

John wanted to see more, as much more as he could. In Scotland, London had seemed like a distant place. But after he had been in London for a few years, and had listened to the tales that seamen told in bars, he felt the pull of adventure.

As usual, the empire was at war with France, and there was, as usual, a desperate need for surgeons. In 1761 John applied for a surgeon's commission and sailed with a contingent being sent to help defend a strategic fortress on Belle-Île, off the coast of France.

For almost two years, as the English and the French struggled on land and at sea, John sewed up wounds and amputated limbs in the Belle-Île Army hospital.

Conditions at the hospital were very good, for the times. There was a matron, and nurses to care for the wounded. There were almost enough doctors and surgeons to go around. But the hospital, as field hospitals had always been, was largely a place for dying.

The cannon and the musket were still new and terrifying weapons, and the damage they did was hideous. A piece of flying shrapnel could lay open the belly of a running soldier, and he would trip on his own intestines. A musket ball could enter the body, glance from rib to rib, and tear a chest apart. A cannon could reduce a man to a fine splatter of blood and bone.

The patients John saw, of course, were those who lived long enough to get to the hospital: They had broken bones, musket ball wounds in the soft tissues, and blown-off limbs. But they weren't necessarily more fortunate than their comrades who died on the field.

John and his fellow surgeons had no idea why the area around a wound began to putrefy in a few days, but they knew it did. First the mangled flesh grew red and inflamed, and pus began to ooze from it. Later the tissue turned gray, with a greenish tint, and tiny gas-filled blisters appeared. Finally, as the gangrene climbed up the limb toward the body, the flesh behind it turned black. In that manner, a musket wound to the hand or foot could often prove fatal.

In the beginning, the victim screamed a lot. Later, as the gangrene crept toward the vital organs, a merciful fever set in.

Medicine was useless against gangrene, but sometimes

John's knife could save the victim. If John saw the soldier soon enough, and the wound was minor enough, the patient could be held down while John cut away the bruised flesh around the wound. Sometimes, then, the wound healed before the gangrene could set in. And if that didn't work, amputation high above the gangrene sometimes stopped its deadly advance.

John became very adept at amputations. On a good day, he could lop off a leg in thirty seconds. The screams echoed down the dark hallways and there, unlike on the battlefield, there were no cannon to drown them out.

Though he hadn't been much affected by the silent corpses in his brother's anatomy laboratory, the living screams were different. They moved him so deeply that, in an attempt to lessen the suffering around him, he actually resorted to books. When he found them unhelpful, he began collecting notes on his own experiences and, slowly, a manuscript grew. By the time he returned to London he carried with him a treatise on the treatment of gunshot wounds and the deadly infections that followed.

But by that time the war was over and England, finally at peace, wasn't very interested in battlefield medicine. The manuscript gathered dust.

John opened an office in Golden Square and set about the slow process of building a practice. At first, because of his well-known interest in corpses, business was very slow.

He is, they whispered, *a ghoul. He cuts up bodies in his house. In his house! Near the office where, he says, he'll treat you. Either way, you're business for him.*

Yet he was also a jolly little man, fully capable of sharing a mug of ale with his patients. If you didn't know ahead of time that he was a ghoul, why, you could actually find yourself liking him. And if you couldn't pay, he'd trust you. And if you didn't get around to paying before you got sick again, you could go back to him with confidence that he would have completely forgotten the debt. And you could see, when he examined you, that he was really interested. And . . . somehow . . . his patients seemed to do better than other doctors' patients.

So while it was true that if you died he would probably turn ghoul and dismember your remains, well, until then you would get better.

Even his fellow surgeons were impressed with John Hunter's remarkable success with patients. As time passed he was admitted to the corporation of surgeons and elected a surgeon at St. George's Hospital. His practice, which had grown slowly at first, finally prospered.

As a result, he had the money to invest in curiosity. And now, unlike during his anatomy days, he didn't have to ask his brother's permission to save things. He quickly became well known to those who dealt in the exotica of the empire.

An ostrich?

There's an ostrich in London? Where? How much?

The more his lust was apparent, the higher the price. If there was an ostrich in London, then John Hunter had to have it, he just had to. And, at a ruinous cost, he did.

Also a zebra.

In 1767 he purchased two acres at nearby Earl's Court, so that he could house his exotic fowl, rabbits, opossums, hedgehogs, jackals, pigs, and water buffalo.

For exercise he had purchased a small bull that he would goad into charging him, and then he would wrestle it to the ground. Once the bull got the upper hand and would have killed him, had not a servant stepped in and distracted the animal. John Hunter dusted himself off and laughed. If you were to live fully, you had to take risks. There was more truth in a brush with death than in all the books ever written.

He collected dead animals as well as live ones, and his home was soon bursting with the skeletons of strange creatures from places like India and black Africa. With the instinct that Charles Darwin would one day carry to its logical conclusion, he studied the animals he had, trying to deduce the relationships between them and their environments.

You could tell what kind of things an animal ate, for instance, by looking at its teeth. Plant eaters had flat teeth, for grinding. Carnivores had sharp ones, for ripping and tearing.

Teeth, in particular, fascinated him. He thought about writing a book on teeth, but books, well, what were books? Books were dead plants, pounded beyond recognition. . . .

Still. He was maturing, and was learning that the obvious facts could sometimes obscure important, but more subtle, truths. The world wasn't in books, it was true. But could it be understood without them? Perhaps, one day, he would write. . . .

For the moment he didn't write much about what he was doing, but he talked plenty, and the stories passed among the gentlemen of the Royal Academy. Increasingly, the gentlemen scientists who gathered there sought to meet John Hunter.

John happily received them and escorted them through the private museum that, by now, occupied most of the space in his home. As he pulled out skeleton after skeleton, he explained what truths of nature could be deduced from each one.

He had human skeletons, too, and the visitors were always awed by them. But, sadly, John had to admit that this collection was grievously incomplete.

What it lacked was a giant.

Some men, as everyone knew, were born giants. They

were rare, but there was one alive, even now, in London. His name was O'Brien and he was more than seven feet tall.

Seven feet! Imagine!

The average, in 18th-century England, was closer to five feet.

John's craving for a giant's skeleton led him to approach O'Brien directly. John wasn't one to dance around a point, and he pointed out to O'Brien that, whereas he was growing old and would soon have no need . . .

O'Brien listened, his eyes growing larger and larger as the message sank in. This man, this jolly little ghoul, had taken a liking to his bones!

"Only after you die," John explained. He would remove the flesh, he said, and . . .

O'Brien backed away, not taking his eyes from the ghoul.

"Get out of here! Leave me alone!"

The stupidity of the human race, John Hunter was repeatedly forced to conclude, was infinite. He just didn't understand O'Brien's reaction. What was so important about a skeleton, anyway? Did O'Brien think he'd need it in heaven? John resolved to keep his eye on the giant, and to bide his time. He made certain that the body snatchers of London, with whom he maintained close contact, all knew of his desire.

Patience didn't come easily to John Hunter, but he understood that occasionally it was necessary. So he waited until, inevitably, a man came to his office and informed him that the giant was sick. The informant left, still surprised at the generous size of the reward.

John acted immediately, summoning a trusted . . . associate . . . named Howison. Howison listened carefully to the instructions, and gratefully accepted the large pile of coins that the surgeon proffered.

While it was true that the giant was ill, he wasn't yet bedridden. He left his home frequently to take in the fresh air, to go to the market, and to attend church. He soon noticed the man who followed him at a distance.

The ghoul, O'Brien's friends agreed. *The ghoul wants your bones. He makes no secret of it.*

O'Brien knew death was coming, and with God to give him courage he had faced the fact. But the vision of his flesh being stripped from his bones by the ghoul, and of his bones dancing from a hook in a trophy case, was more than O'Brien could accept.

Desperately, he went to the undertaker with all the money he could scrape together.

After he died, he told the undertaker, he wanted his body to be under constant guard until a suitably large lead coffin could be obtained. When the coffin was ready, his body should be placed in it, taken to sea, and dropped into the deep. There it would be forever out of reach of the ghouls. When the undertaker swore to do as instructed, the giant gave him his savings. Thus protected, the giant died in peace in 1763.

John Hunter knew of the event within the hour, of course, and began making inquiries. When he learned the body was under constant guard and would be buried at sea, he wasn't dismayed.

The question was, who were the guards? And where did the guards go to drink? Howison, grateful in advance for the generous gratuity he always received, already had the answer.

John immediately left for the tavern.

Legends grow around such transactions as occurred that day, and legend says that John, his eagerness plain to see, immediately offered the guards fifty pounds for the corpse.

Fifty pounds was a fortune in those days, a year's pay.

The guards would have sold their trust for much less. But John, enraptured by the vision of the giant's skeleton hanging in his collection, didn't see the surprise on their faces.

The guards said they would have to step outside and discuss the matter and so, while John waited impatiently, they disappeared.

The conversation outside must be imagined. Fifty pounds for one corpse? The question was, what kind of a fool would pay fifty pounds for one bloody corpse? The answer was obvious. A rich fool.

Soon the guards were back, playing it coy. John Hunter, in his impatient lust, was no match for them and, legend says, he paid the princely sum of five hundred pounds for the cadaver.

To him, the price was irrelevant. What was money for, if not to spend on things to enlighten the mind and satiate the curiosity?

It came as no surprise to scientific London when, that night, some person or persons overpowered three guards and snatched the body of the Irish giant, O'Brien. Soon the curious gentlemen scientists were coming in twos and threes to visit Dr. Hunter, the surgeon, and to inspect the seven-foot skeleton he had hung from a hook in the room above his office.

It was apparent to the men from the Royal Society that John Hunter was something special, and that he was bringing a new rationality to medicine. In 1767 they made him a member.

Many Londoners, of course, failed to appreciate Dr. Hunter's ghoulish behavior, and mobs occasionally gathered outside his home. He dealt with them by barring the doors and shutters and continuing to work. Lynch mobs have a short attention span, he reasoned, and they eventually got bored and went somewhere to get drunk.

The trouble with the world, as he saw it, was ignorance, the kind of ignorance epitomized by the mob. They
looked, but refused to see. They were blinded by sacred
ideas out of the medieval past. The obvious was lost on
them.

Such ignorance was not, unfortunately, confined to the
mob. Some of John's own fellow surgeons and doctors
were sometimes guilty of dramatic stupidity . . . about the
pox, for instance. As much as John tried to explain that it
was two manifestations of the same disease, some experts
refused to understand what was being explained to them.
They persisted in believing that the pox was two distinct
diseases.

He tried to be patient with them, because they were, in
theory at least, his peers. He tried to be patient, but patience was not among his strengths. Finally, fed up, he
resolved to end the matter once and for all.

As the farmers back in Scotland might say, it was the
sort of thing that only a ghoul would think to do, and he
did it on a Friday.

A patient with the pox stood before him, his pants
down to his knees. A tiny drop of yellowish liquid hung
from the tip of his penis. It was a classic case, in John's
view, of the pox attacking the soft, wet tissue and producing, naturally, a wet discharge.

John stared at the drop of pus, thinking. It was a classic
case, a perfect case, an opportunity not to be passed up.
To prove that the pox was a single disease, all he needed
to show was that the pus from this patient, a "wet" case,
could produce a chancre, or a "dry" case, in another penis.

John only had one healthy penis handy, so he used it.

Carefully, while the patient stood before him, he took
the droplet on a lancet and transferred it to the glans of his
own penis. Then, through the droplet, he stabbed himself
with the lancet. For good measure, he stabbed himself

again. He squeezed the small cuts open, so that the liquid miasma of the pox could take hold.

That done, he replaced his own penis in his pants and turned his attention back to the patient. He gave the man a bit of mercury and instructed him to rub it into his thighs. If he did so, the doctor promised, the discharge would go away in a couple of weeks. The secondary symptoms would come later, but in time they, too, would go away.

Thoughtfully, John watched the man leave his office. Then he went back to work.

There were absolutely no surprises in what happened. That Sunday John confided in his notebook that his penis had begun tingling in a way that was really rather pleasant. There was also a redness where the lancet had pierced the skin. By the following Tuesday there were two little pimplelike chancres.

They were firm, like the tissues they arose from. A runny disease had produced a dry disease, proving, once and for all, that while it had many forms, the pox was but one disease.

John had taken, in recent years, to writing things down on paper, and even occasionally publishing them, and this was certainly worth committing to print. Shortly a paper was published and, because it was written by Dr. Hunter, it received the immediate and respectful attention of England's doctors. They read the details of the experiment, shook their heads, and conceded the argument. Dr. Hunter was correct. Pox was a single disease.

Having proved his point, John remained caught up in the enigma of the pox. Now that he watched it develop in his own body, he had to marvel at its complexity. He toyed with it, curious as to its response.

He dropped a bit of acid on one of chancres and it dropped off, but it was replaced by another one just like it.

He rubbed some mercury into his thighs and the chancres disappeared. He wrote in his notebook that they left two small dimples that retained a bluish cast for a long time.

There the matter rested until, nine months later, he developed a sore throat. By examining himself in a mirror, he located a small ulcer on a tonsil.

Secondary pox?

He rubbed some mercury into his thigh, and the ulcer went away.

Three months later he got a skin rash and treated it with mercury, but this time he was very careful not to give himself enough to make the symptoms vanish entirely. He found that, by toying with the amount of mercury, he could make the rash and the sore throat come and go at will.

That was interesting, he thought. The pox might be one disease but it also had two definite stages. That should be telling him something.

He worried at the problem, but found no ready answer. Finally, frustrated and bored, he rubbed a massive dose of mercury into his thigh and the symptoms, he wrote in his notebook, disappeared for good. John went on to other, more important things.

As the years passed, then a decade, then another, John Hunter's studies of animal and human bodies opened a new frontier in medicine. The dike broke in 1771 with a treatise on the natural history of human teeth, which was followed by a paper the next year on the stomach's curious ability to digest itself after death. Suddenly John Hunter's writing exploded into the later half of the 18th century.

The impact of his work was related only tangentially to the facts he presented. The Hunterian tradition, as it would later be called, didn't rest on John Hunter's study of whales, or his approach to the treatment of gunshot wounds, or his observations concerning the descent of the

testicles in young males. The Hunterian tradition was em-
bodied in the sheer force of his relentless curiosity, and if
his answers were sometimes wrong, it didn't matter. All
answers led to more questions, and in those answers the
truth could be seen and the record corrected. It was a phi-
losophy before which Mother Nature seemed to become
strangely compliant.

Curiosity was the light of the new age, the kernel of
science, and sometimes the song of a siren.

A striped dog with a pouch like a kangaroo? Really?
How much?

Who owns it?

Take me to him!

John lived for years on Golden Square, putting off moving as long as he could. But the inevitable day came when
the closets were filled with skeletons and the shelves were
lined with specimens in jars. He had to either move or
throw something away, and so he moved.

The new house on Leicester Square was far larger than
the old one, and it had plenty of room in the back for
expansion. To make certain he wouldn't be cramped, he
also purchased the house behind it, on Castle Street. That
did the trick, except . . . John contemplated the four tall
drawing-room windows in the main house.

They were nice, and they would let in a lot of light, but
. . . the world was full of fools like the Irish giant
O'Brien, and fools often carried torches and ropes, and ran
together in mobs.

While the workmen attached heavy shutters that could
swing closed and seal off the windows in front, John paced
the empty houses. There was room, much more room
than on Golden Square. But still not enough.

When he was finished, the house in back had been converted to utilitarian purposes, such as dissections and specimen preparation.

Between the houses, and adjoining both, Hunter constructed a huge building. On the bottom floor there was a lecturing theater and a meeting room.

The most important area of all was on the second floor of that building. The museum was fifty-two feet long and twenty-eight feet wide, lit naturally from the top. Lovingly, he arranged his specimens in it and marked each one with a neatly printed label. He had a special place for O'Brien's skeleton.

His new home pleased him, and the friends who called on him there were quick and intelligent, and knew the sacred power of questions. In the evenings they talked and speculated, and during the day John treated an increasingly wealthy practice. Even the queen sent him gifts. It was a perfect way to grow old, except . . .

John was made of flesh and bone, an organism designed to sustain life only so long, and no longer. The time was approaching when he, too, would lie on the marble slab. He knew it, and he didn't need the gray hair to remind him. The pain in his chest told him. In the beginning the pain was neither severe nor frequent, but as an anatomist he couldn't ignore the sign.

John Hunter knew only one way to deal with death, and that was to ignore it completely. But there was an urgency to life now, and a deep need to commit things to paper. He concentrated on writing, dissecting, teaching, treating patients, and concocting ever newer and better questions with his fellow ghouls.

But by his sixtieth birthday the pains in his chest had begun to strike at the very worst time, in the midst of excitement. That was very inconvenient and had cost him an increasingly large number of arguments. When the pain had passed, all he could do was grimace weakly at his opponent.

At least, he said, he didn't have a usual heart. It must be very remarkable indeed, to cause such pain. It would be an interesting heart, he imagined, and would fascinate whoever pulled it from his chest.

"When I die," he commanded, "take out my heart and put it in a bottle."

His friends stood by, awkward in the face of such talk, and counseled patience, temperance, moderation, calmness. John recognized their advice as reasonable . . . it was, in fact, precisely the advice he would give a patient under similar circumstances. He respected the advice, and thanked his friends for it, and then ignored it completely.

The inevitable happened in 1793. He was embroiled in a loud quarrel, as usual, with the hospital board. He was making the broad point, as he was wont to do, that the board was composed of as representative a band of nincompoops as could be found anywhere in London. Suddenly, at the peak of his argument, his hands rose to his chest and he sank to the floor.

Slowly, as friends and adversaries knelt around him, his fingernails turned from pink to blue, his eyes rolled up in his head, and he died. A chair was found to bear his corpse home to Leicester Square.

Now, in the dissecting room, an assistant honed the knives against a steel rod, moving them expertly back and forth, snick, snick, snick. The naked form that was no longer John Hunter lay on the slab.

The senior ghoul called for a knife. He made the Y incision smoothly, slicing from each nipple to the sternum in the center of the chest, then down to the pubic bone. The white fat of the belly, testimony to too much beer and food, pulled open of its own weight. The intestines shone wetly in the body cavity.

Working together, the ghouls removed the slippery bowels, along with the kidneys, pancreas, and spleen, and placed them in pans for later study. The liver, somewhat altered by alcohol consumption, followed.

When the abdominal cavity was empty, the ghouls moved on to the chest. The ribs cracked loudly as they parted. The men in the room had been his friends and students, but there were no visible emotions. John, while alive, had always refused to attend the funerals of friends on the grounds that it was ignoble to bow and scrape and sob in the presence of some corpse. Emotions now, at his autopsy, would be unfitting to the Hunterian tradition.

The ghouls reached their bloody hands into the chest cavity and grasped the heart. The knife cut cleanly through the great vessels and the organ was free. They carried it to a nearby table and sliced it open. The ghouls passed the heart from hand to hand. Each examined it carefully, shook his head, and passed it on.

The day would come, in the remote future, when beneficiaries of the Hunterian tradition would discover, by rigorous observation and pugnacious curiosity, that the pox was in fact two diseases—John Hunter had been wrong. But it would be a century before microscopes focused on the gonococcus bacterium and the syphilis spirochete. Only then did it become clear that a patient could have both at once, and pass on both . . . or only one. They would discover that the form of the pox that had seemed the worst to John Hunter, the wet one that caused so much discomfort, was really the less dangerous. It was gonorrhea.

The other one, the one that produced the chancre, was syphilis. As scientists would later come to understand, mercury would kill a few of the spirochetes . . . but never enough to do more than mask the symptoms. They would also learn that syphilis had not two stages, but three. In its third stage it could attack a variety of organs, including the heart, brain, spinal cord—and aorta. This made it by far the more dangerous of the two diseases.

But the early pathologists, only a few years removed from grave robbing, knew nothing of this. As they passed the heart from hand to hand they observed, in passing, that the aorta seemed somewhat enlarged.

But in the year 1793, in an era when the pox was rampant, an enlarged aorta was a common finding—not associated, in anyone's mind, with the pox. John Hunter's heart, as even John Hunter would have had to agree, was wholly unremarkable, not the kind of heart to save in a jar. The pathology report listed the cause of his heart disease as unknown, and the heart itself plopped softly into the waiting bucket to be discarded. John Hunter's life ended, as it had been lived, with a question.

He had been a special man, who had heard the siren as a child. She mesmerized him, fascinated him, captured him, and blessed him with the bright questioning force that would shape the future. But so great was the legend that surrounded him, so unassailable was any conclusion connected with his name, that it would be a hundred years before medical scientists would have the temerity to question his work on the pox and discover the magnitude of his error, and that he had died of tertiary syphilis—and by his own hand. Only then would it be known that the siren had led him in the end, in dark and ironic ignorance, to his death.

And as for the skeleton of the giant O'Brien, it hangs today in the museum of the Royal College of Surgeons in London, grinning its mute testimony that the forces of curiosity are more powerful than those of fear.

THE SAD TALE OF
LAUGHING GAS

Horace Wells was born into the American Dream in 1815, the year that the first steam-driven warship, the USS *Fulton*, was launched. He spent his boyhood in the arms of Vermont Protestantism, learned to read the Bible under the strict tutelage of his mother, and came, by the osmosis of childhood, to understand the divinity of Accomplishment.

Inventors like James Watt and Michael Faraday were set before him to admire, as soldiers in the war for progress. When he was two, construction began on the Erie Canal. When he was three, the steamship *Savannah* crossed the Atlantic in an incredible twenty-six days. When he was six, sound was first recorded. When he was eight, Charles Babbage began the first of his many attempts to build a machine that would add and subtract. When he was twelve, Josef Ressel invented the first ship's propeller. When he was fourteen, the patent office issued papers for the first typewriter. It was only natural that Horace would grow to expect similar contributions from himself.

Horace's adolescent vision of his future had many romantic aspects, but the romanticism stopped at the ledger book. While it was necessary for him to make a contribution to the world as an inventor, it wouldn't do to be a

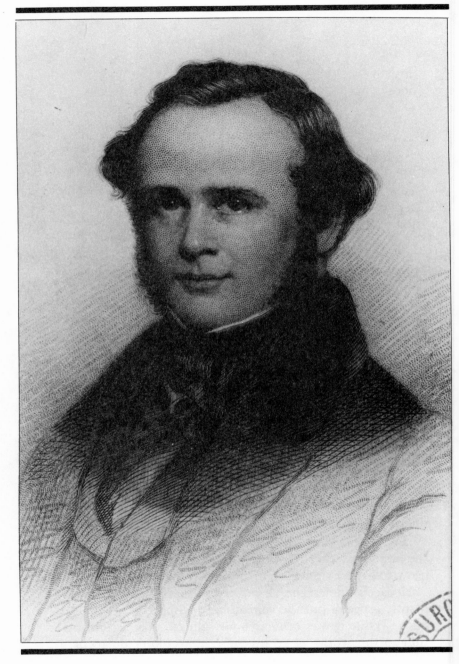

DR. HORACE WELLS

starving inventor. He knew early in his life that he must choose a profession—a humanitarian profession, of course —that would serve to financially underwrite his ambitions. It would also have to be a profession that was in need of someone like him, so that he could contribute to it, and perhaps achieve fame and fortune in that manner.

His ambitions were, as he had been taught they should be, without limitation. But in the prosaic world of reality, there were certain courses denied to him. He thought of medicine, and yearned for the wealth and respect it brought, but he couldn't afford medical school. He considered law, but not for long. Law was full of cobwebs, and law schools were almost as expensive as medical schools. Engineering had its appeal, but it took forever to become an engineer. And then there was dentistry. . . .

Dentistry.

As he applied himself to the demands of high school, he thought the problem over again and again, and it always came down to dentistry. In the first place dentists, like doctors, helped people. Dentists befriended suffering humanity in the most direct way.

In addition, dentistry was a secure profession. When times were good, dentists pulled teeth. When times were bad, they pulled teeth. And the patient, by the time he got to the dentist, was in a poor bargaining position, so a dentist could demand, and get, payment in cash. Beforehand. A dental practice, prudently managed, could be a source of wealth as well as respect.

The price was right, as well. There was no school of dentistry anywhere in the Americas, and no laws to prevent an aspiring dentist from buying the necessary tools, hanging out a shingle, and going into practice. Many did just that, though Horace didn't look with favor on that option. It would be better, for the patients, to serve first as an apprentice.

So it was that in 1824, as high school graduation neared, nineteen-year-old Horace applied for, and got, an apprenticeship with a dentist in Boston. As soon as the commencement ceremonies were over he packed his bags and left Vermont in hot pursuit of fame, fortune, and service to humanity.

Horace had chosen wisely, in the sense that dentistry was indeed a fallow field for innovation. While the dexterity required of a dentist wasn't to be disdained, the equipment and practices then in use were in obvious need of improvement. False teeth rarely fit properly. The solder used for metal bridgework set up a galvanic reaction in the mouth that caused the patient's breath to stink with the stench of the grave. And the pain . . .

In imagining himself a dentist, the idealistic young man from Vermont had dreamed of helping people, had reveled in the gratitude he would certainly receive from his patients, had thought long on the matter of profits. That much he could understand from afar. The fact that a dentist must inflict pain had somehow never intruded on his reveries.

Like most people, he had avoided thinking of pain at all, and when he did, his mind automatically came to rest on the specter of the surgeon.

John Hunter's brother William had once characterized surgeons as "savages armed with knives," and the basic condition of their practice hadn't changed in the new century. The surgeon and his burly assistants still arrived, like the undertaker and priest, at a time of terrible crisis, and they weren't deterred by either curses or screamed pleas. The fact that a surgeon was called at all was a tribute to the powerful, and sometimes terrible, human will to live.

Most people dealt with the subject of pain as they always had, looking to their faith for the strength to endure it. Hadn't the Lord told Eve that "in pain thou shalt bring forth children"? Pain built character, they said. It cleansed you and made you humble before God.

Though schools of surgery sought to make their students as callous as possible, occasional surgeons nevertheless found themselves distracted by all the screaming and struggling, and over the centuries many attempts were made to alleviate the agony. Alcohol was tried, but the surgeons found that the patient who appeared to be dead drunk nevertheless woke up as soon as the knife touched his flesh. Ancient writings indicated that an extract of mandrake could help, but the surgeons of the 19th century found it wholly ineffective. Hypnotism was tried and that, too, failed.

One French surgeon experimented with narcotics and, for his trouble, was accused of witchcraft. In Germany, F.W.A. Sertürner proposed morphine for pain but was so derided for his efforts that he abandoned his experiments and concentrated on more socially acceptable goals. He eventually won fame for improving the design of breech-loading weapons.

But while surgeons were the most feared, surgery was really very infrequent. During one 5-year period in the middle 1800s, Massachusetts General Hospital recorded only 184 operations, 3 per month, and most of those were superficial. Frustrated surgeons developed elaborate surgical procedures to carry them into the chest and abdomen, and frequently tried them out on cadavers. But not even the most egotistical surgeon would attempt to perform such delicate operations on a shrieking, squirming patient. When an appendix swelled and burst, the patient belonged not to the surgeon but to the undertaker.

So while everyone knew someone who knew someone who had had a leg, arm, or breast amputated, a merciful

few actually benefited—if that is the correct word—from
the knife. The surgeon was a faraway, terrible, almost
mythical creature who preyed, one hoped, on someone
else.

The dentist was a different matter. Almost everybody
had a few rotten teeth. Sweets were given to children, but
few adults dared to bite into chocolates. Periodically, the
rotten teeth ached.

Prayer helped, some said. Also a bag of ice on the jaw.
If you could endure the pain long enough, you could out-
last it and it would go away. Sometimes it did and, then
again, sometimes it didn't.

By the time the victims finally arrived at the office
where Horace Wells served as apprentice, their faces were
haggard from days of agony, and they had been reduced,
emotionally, to childhood. They were usually accompanied by several family members who would serve a
soothing and comforting function during the ordeal to
come.

Some of the patients arrived with a facade of bravado,
but it fell as soon as they were seated in the terrible chair.

The dentist's first task was to peer into the mouth to
determine which of the many rotten teeth was causing the
pain. After it had been identified, the dentist reached into
the mouth with a pair of long-handled forceps.

At this moment it was Horace's function as apprentice
to reach out and grab the patient.

Sharply, the dentist pulled up on the handles, and the
tooth rocked backward in its socket . . .

Aaaaaaagh!

. . . and then forward . . .

Ahhhhhhhh!

. . . backward . . .

Owwwwwwwwwwwwwww!

At this stage of the procedure the patient typically

changed his mind and tried to grab for the forceps, at the same time sliding down into the chair, howling. It was Horace's job as apprentice to keep the arms down. He put his strength into it.

Yah! Yah! Yaaaaaaaaaaaaaaaaaaaaaaaaaaaaaaaaaaaa . . .

When all went well there was a distinctive crunching noise as the roots broke free from the jawbone. With a jerk of the dentist's biceps the tooth came out, followed by the last, and usually loudest, shriek.

The dentist stepped back smartly, tooth held high in the forceps. As the patient collapsed forward, his hands reaching for his mouth, Horace deftly put a pan in his lap. That protected the clothing from the gush of blood.

But often all did not go well and the crunching sound was of a different sort, more like the sound of a pecan breaking. That was the tooth collapsing inward and disintegrating under the pressure of the forceps. Then, well . . . that was a pity. But the roots had to come out.

The dentist had special instruments for that—drills, chisels, and small sharp knives. The patient never cooperated but he did eventually become exhausted and the screams died to whimpers, which made it easier. It was all routine for the dentist.

But somehow it didn't become routine for Horace. Other people's pain became commonplace in his life, and he endured it with them, but it never became routine. Sometimes he ran his tongue uneasily around his mouth and found the familiar cavities that would one day force him to sit in the chair himself. He identified too much with his patients for pain ever to become routine, and despite his upbringing he could never convince himself it was good for the soul.

In that sense he didn't have a natural talent for his chosen field, but he made up for it with determination and effort and he survived the apprenticeship. In 1836, the year he reached the age of his majority, his name, with the honorific "Dr." in front of it, appeared above the door of a small office in Hartford, Connecticut. He was finally on his way.

He had chosen Hartford, the state capital, because it seemed in need of another dentist. In that he was correct, and his growing practice was aided as well by his distaste for pain. Though Horace hurt his patients as much as his competitors, his regret and compassion was apparent to his customers and they passed along a recommendation to their friends. Dr. Wells was the dentist to see, assuming you had tried everything else and absolutely had to see a dentist. He would even give you credit, if you needed it.

Within two years the young dentist had a practice large enough to allow him to think about marriage. And that, of course, required a girl.

There was only one place to find a proper wife, and that was in church. Discreetly, he began to let his eyes lift up from the hymnal and survey the eligible females. While the sermons droned on, he cataloged them. Then, one by one, he rejected them as too fat, too thin, or too tall, or too short, until there was only one left.

Step two was to ascertain her name and address, which he did with a little detective work. Finally, at home, he set out ink and paper, and picked up his pen.

"Dear Elizabeth . . ."

Was that too informal? Familiar?

He crumpled the page, threw it in the wastebasket, and took a new sheet. Eventually that sheet, too, was reduced to a crumpled ball, and was followed by the next, and the next, and the next.

The final version was dated several days later, March 5, 1838. Horace's shaking hands folded the missive, put it in an envelope, and sealed it. For a handsome tip a child took the letter and put it into Elizabeth's hands.

The tortured, formal phrases testified to the agony of their creation, but they befitted a suitor at the opening of the Victorian age.

". . . Would it be in accordance with your wishes to become more familiarly acquainted with me? . . . Excuse me for being explicit. . . . Are there circumstances which preclude the possibility of this proposed acquaintance ever resulting in a more intimate connection than that of brother and sister in Christ?"

It was, however stilted, a love letter. Elizabeth was impressed and wrote back the next day.

"Dear Dr. Wells, sir . . . I am . . . prepared to say . . . that to cultivate a farther acquaintance with you would be agreeable to my wishes. . . ."

After an awkward series of visits, matrimony was broached and accepted. The wedding was on July 8.

That accomplished, Horace turned his energies to perfecting his first invention, a device that allowed one to sift through coal dust and retrieve the burnable clinkers without getting one's hands dirty. The next year his wife presented him with a son and the U.S. government issued him his first patent.

In Horace's fastidious mind his brainchild was an important contribution. He assumed that the world would beat a path to his door, buying endless copies of the device that would allow them to keep their hands clean while saving pennies and even dollars on unburned clinkers. He waited impatiently for the income to begin to flow into his bank account.

His confidence was high, and it dwindled slowly, but by the time his son was a toddler Horace had been forced to realize that the clinker retriever was a dud. The acceptance of that truth was bitter, but it was followed by a new wave of confidence. If at first you don't succeed, his mother had taught him, then you must try, and try again.

Perhaps he could become a well-known author. The more he thought about the idea the more it suited him, and he set about producing a small, scholarly book entitled *An Essay on Teeth: Comprising a Brief Description of Their Formation, Disease, and Proper Treatment.* The book was published in 1841.

By that year the dentistry practice had grown large enough that Wells could begin accepting apprentices. For the first, he chose a young man named William T. G. Morton. Though in the best of possible worlds Wells would have preferred someone less . . . well, brash than Morton, the apprentice was in all other respects satisfactory.

Morton soon proved susceptible to his teacher's inventive visions, and the two began trying to invent something together. They finally settled on the problem of bridgework odor. It was produced, they decided, by a chemical reaction caused by the silver solder that was commonly used in bridgework. The solution would be to find a different kind of solder.

By this time Wells, now in his mid-twenties, had already laid the foundation for achieving his ambition. He was a successful if not yet wealthy dentist who drew his patients from the aristocracy of Hartford. Wells even treated the governor and his family. His profession was a stable platform upon which he would build.

Stable . . . yet his profession was not really a pleasant one. The incessant suffering still depressed him. He even complained to his friends, wishing aloud that there was some way, some method of stopping the pain. Perhaps one day . . .

In the meantime there was success on the invention front. Wells and Morton had graduated from the apprentice-master relationship, and as the two worked late into the night, pursuing their dream of solderless bridgework, they became first allies and then close friends.

When the process was perfected, they were ecstatic. It was, they convinced one another, their key to a prosperous future. The only problem left to be solved was that of marketing and that, they were certain, would be simple. As soon as the world heard about the odorless dental plate, why, they would both be rich.

The invention was too important, they told one another, to unveil in a little backwater place like Hartford. They decided to go instead to Boston, the intellectual capital of the world. Wells closed down his dental office in Hartford, packed his bags, kissed his wife and son goodbye, and set off, with Morton, for the big city.

Once there they put an advertisement in the paper and sat back to await the influx of customers. But no one came.

The friendship between Wells and Morton had seemed rock solid in Hartford, but in the face of failure the bond dissolved. The two quarreled and Morton walked out, resolving to give up dentistry entirely and enroll instead in medical school. Horace repacked his things and returned to Hartford in defeat, to reopen his office.

So in 1844, with Horace Wells one year shy of the watershed age of thirty, it was a quietly desperate man who opened the newspaper and saw the advertisement.

A grand exhibition of the effects produced by inhaling nitrous oxide, exhilarating or laughing gas!
Will be given at Union Hall this evening (Tuesday),
December 10, 1844.

Twelve young men have volunteered to inhale the gas to commence the entertainment.

Eight strong men are engaged to occupy the front seats to protect those under the influence of the gas from injuring themselves or others. (The gas will be administered only to gentlemen of the first

respectability. The object is to make the entertainment in every
respect a genteel affair.)

Horace looked at the ad. It might be fun. Interesting, that is. It might make him feel better. His Protestant training didn't usually allow for entertainment but, according to the advertisement, this wasn't exactly entertainment. It was more like a scientific lecture, and there was certainly no sin in science. Besides, it might do him good to forget his troubles for a while. Elizabeth agreed.

Wells arrived at the Union Hall, bought his ticket and went inside. It was almost time for the show to start.

He stood for a moment in the rear, his eyes adjusting to the light. The hall was about half full. As a man walked on stage and the crowd grew quiet and attentive, Horace slipped into a seat apart from the others.

The man introduced himself as Professor Gardner Colton. He spoke with an exaggerated scientific phrasing that seemed oh so precise, while making nothing clear. There was just enough plain English to ensure that the audience got the gist of it.

The professor had a mysterious gas that he carried around in inflatable bladders, and if you breathed it, he said, you'd act funny. The professor got very quickly to the meat of the program, which was asking for volunteers.

The first man to stand up was one Horace knew well, a drugstore clerk named Samuel Cooley. Horace watched as Cooley mounted the stage and sat down in a wooden chair. The professor put a tube under Samuel's nose and Samuel breathed deeply, as instructed.

The change was almost instantaneous. Cooley jumped up from his chair and started shadowboxing with an imaginary opponent . . . imaginary, that is, until someone in the audience laughed. Cooley stopped his shadowboxing, his eyes searching for the source of laughter. In a flash,

Cooley bounded toward the man, momentarily eluding the eight strong men and in the process banging his shin on a table.

Cooley's shin hit the wood so hard, and made such a loud thwack, that Horace, the gentle dentist, winced in sympathy. But Cooley, his mind aflame with gas and emotion, continued his charge as though nothing had happened. In the confusion he reached the aisle before the effects of the gas wore off. The anger on his face changed to puzzlement and, as quickly as it had come, the crisis was over. The audience roared. Red-faced, Cooley slunk up the aisle and collapsed into a seat next to Horace.

As the professor led the next volunteer onto the stage, Horace leaned over and expressed his sympathy about the injured shin.

Shin? Cooley asked. Injured shin? What injured shin?

At Wells's insistence, Cooley leaned over and rolled up his pants leg. Sure enough, there was a fast-swelling lump. Surprised, Cooley touched it and grimaced. It hurt now, he said . . . but at the time he hadn't felt a thing.

Horace gazed at him in disbelief, then turned his attention back to the stage, where another upright Hartford citizen had just begun to laugh like an idiot.

Laughing gas, the professor called it.

Horace's mind worked furiously.

Laughing gas.

What was laughing gas?

After the demonstration was over, as the crowd filed out of the auditorium, Wells hung back until all the others had gone. Then he approached Professor Colton, who was leaning on the lectern.

Colton was friendly and, his audience now gone, was willing to discuss the gas in detail. It was called nitrous oxide, he told the inquisitive dentist. Colton explained that, with the backing of P. T. Barnum, he was making a good living going around the country and presenting "scientific lectures" with it. It was a wonderful scheme. . . . People loved nothing better than to see their fellowmen making fools of themselves.

Wells listened carefully. The mention of P. T. Barnum made him pause. It wasn't exactly a scientific connection but, still . . . the gas was real. Wells had seen it work with his own two eyes. He offered a proposition and Professor Colton thought about it. Yes, he said in a moment, he would be amenable to cooperating in an experiment.

Wells left the hall, his mind spinning with possibilities. He felt lonely with his idea, and he wished Morton were there. He needed someone to talk to.

As he walked toward home, a thought occurred to him and he altered his course. In a few minutes he arrived at the home of another former student, Dr. John Riggs, who had set up his own practice in Hartford. Riggs, happy to see his old teacher, opened the door and let him in. Wells was no sooner inside than he blurted out his brainstorm.

Riggs was skeptical. Painless extractions would be wonderful, but . . . how would you pull a tooth while a patient laughed uproariously?

Obviously you couldn't, Horace conceded. So you'd have to administer more gas than the professor had. The patient would have to be the equivalent of dead drunk.

But what if the gas made the patient more dead than drunk?

Horace dismissed the problem. It wouldn't. He was certain.

Skeptically, Riggs pursued the question more specifically. What if the patient didn't wake up when the tooth was pulled, and he sucked the blood down into his lungs? What then?

Wells thought about that, and didn't have a ready answer. That was a risk, he conceded. He hadn't thought of that and, of course, it precluded trying nitrous oxide on a patient. But that wasn't a problem, because he didn't intend to use a patient anyway. He would use himself, instead. Take the gas first himself. That was where Riggs came in. Riggs would pull a tooth.

Riggs looked at his former teacher, hesitating.

Which tooth? he finally asked.

Horace's inquisitive tongue searched among his cavities and found the largest. Horace opened his mouth and pointed.

Riggs peered into Wells's mouth, examining the tooth. True, it could use extracting. Still. Riggs was uneasy, but he could think of no concrete argument to back up the feeling. Finally, he gave in. He would be at Wells's office first thing in the morning.

Horace walked home, his brain once again aswirl with dreams. He hadn't felt this good since he got the idea for the clinker retriever, or for the solderless bridgework. And this time it was different . . . this time he would succeed. This was an idea that couldn't possibly be overlooked.

Imagine. Extractions without pain!

Imagine a grateful public.

Newspaper writers would want to interview the great Dr. Wells. He would be spoken of even in Boston. It was an intoxicating dream, and Horace arrived home in an expansive mood.

Never had a patient so eagerly awaited the pulling of a tooth. Wells was out of bed and dressed at the crack of dawn, and by the time Riggs arrived at the office, all was in readiness. Samuel Cooley, the pharmacist, showed up a few minutes later, to act as a witness. Finally Professor Colton arrived with a bag of the gas and a friend who had asked to come along and see the show.

As the tiny office became crowded, the observers suddenly remembered Cooley's aggressive behavior the night

before. While Wells waited impatiently, the other partici-
pants discussed their personal safety, finally deciding to
leave the door open. That would provide a quick escape
should Wells turn violent.

The question of observer safety settled, the experiment
quickly got under way. Wells leaned back in the operating
chair, grasping the end of the tubing that led to the professor's gas bladder. There was a wooden spigot on the
end of the tube. Wells turned it, put the opening to his
nose, and breathed deeply.

For a moment he stared into space, his face becoming
pale, then bluish. His eyes rolled up and the lids closed.
His hands fluttered and fell to his lap, dropping the
spigot.

Quickly Dr. Riggs reached out, opened Wells's mouth,
found the tooth, and grasped it with the forceps. He
rocked the forceps sharply, up, then down.

There was no roar of pain, no sound at all except for the
sharp clean crunch of roots separating from jaw. Riggs
stepped back, holding the tooth high.

Almost instantly Wells regained his senses and bent forward to discharge the blood into a pan that someone put in
his lap. When the bleeding had slowed, he stared at the
bloody tooth.

"I didn't even feel a prick," he said softly, his voice full
of wonder.

He accepted the congratulations of Riggs and the spectators and then saw them to the door. When they were all
gone he sat alone in his office, the tooth on the table in
front of him. Again and again his tongue explored the hole
it had left, reassuring him that this was no mere dream.

Imagine, painless extractions! What a profound discovery, what a humanitarian piece of work, what a revolu-
tionary idea. He let the reality percolate through his mind.
The name Horace Wells would be remembered forever!

Suddenly he was on his feet. There was work to do!

*   *   *

In the days and weeks that followed, Wells worked feverishly to develop his idea and to become familiar with the
properties of the gas. In his enthusiasm for the project it
was all he could do to force himself to make time for his
patients, and he let his apprentices do more, perhaps, than
they should have. He neglected his wife and children,
staying at the office and working far into the night with
his retorts, burners, and tubing. What was the best way to
store it, and was it more effective warm or cold? How
much was needed to make the patient dead drunk? And
exactly how drunk was dead drunk?

His mind churned with creative energy until he felt almost . . . drunk?

Hour after hour he sat at his bench, sampling his products, scribbling in his notebook, sometimes wobbling on
his stool, almost losing his balance, nodding off for a moment, waking, breathing deeply of the gas, working,
working, working.

From his upbringing, he knew the dangers of alcohol
and opium, and would never have taken them . . . except,
perhaps, an occasional safe glass of sherry. They could
turn a man into a lunatic, but nitrous oxide wasn't in a
class with them; nitrous oxide was a boon to mankind, a
bright hope in a world shrouded with agony, a buffer
against the veil of tears. He associated his dreams not with
nitrous oxide itself, but with the intoxicating emotional
surge of discovery.

And what dreams they were! Dreams without equal!
Sitting at his bench, inhaling the wonderful gas, he saw
the future with almost startling clarity. Imagine painless
dentistry! Imagine, even, painless surgery! The name
Horace Wells would be in textbooks a thousand years
from now!

He sat for hours, letting the gas seep through his brain,
analyzing it, drifting, coming awake, making notes,

breathing, breathing, breathing, drifting, dreaming.

He would be the most famous dentist of all, and the wealthiest. There would be fine horses, a big house, an infinite supply of new hats for Elizabeth, fame, drifting, drifting, dreaming . . . maybe he would move to Boston . . . drifting, dreaming, breathing . . .

He tried the gas on patients but the results were sometimes more equivocal than they had been with his own extraction. It was puzzling how sometimes . . . sometimes it didn't work. It seemed, somehow, to take different amounts for different people.

When it didn't work, and the patient screamed in agony, it made him impatient, almost angry, and he would experiment some more with himself, drifting, dreaming. It was a mystery why sometimes it failed but . . . his name was Horace Wells, wasn't it? He would figure that out, and correct it. In the meantime, he had . . . he wanted . . . turning the spigot . . . drifting . . . dreaming . . .

In one sense, as a scientist, he should do more preliminary work, and yet, and yet . . . the world needed to know. He needed to make the announcement. His name would be in the newspapers . . . but not in Hartford. Not in Hartford. In Boston! He would unveil the new dream in Boston, before the most famous doctors of all.

Drifting, dreaming, thinking, planning. Yes. Yes. Boston.

Wells wrote to the dean of Harvard surgeons, Dr. John Collins Warren, and Dr. Warren very graciously and promptly replied in the affirmative. He would be pleased, he said, to witness a demonstration. Wells could have the attention of Dr. Warren's medical school class at a convenient date, following a lecture.

Spreading the letter before him on the laboratory bench, Horace read it and read it again. With each reading Dr. Warren sounded more enthusiastic. Horace reached for the gas spigot, opened it, and inhaled deeply. The thing was as good as accomplished. Wells could almost hear the thunderous applause. . . .

He ignored his wife, standing in the background, resentful that he had ceased to notice her. He kissed the child, perfunctorily, on the cheek. His luggage was ready. The bagful of nitrous was safely stowed. Elizabeth blocked his way.

Oh. Of course.

He leaned down and his lips brushed her cheek. Then he pushed by her and was gone.

He arrived in Boston with a day to spare and, unable to contain the news, looked up his old apprentice Morton. Morton was a student at the medical school and was easy to locate.

Morton welcomed his old mentor and then listened, in growing horror, as Wells blurted out his mission. He watched Wells speculatively as the story unfolded.

A gas for pain? Absurd! Had Wells gone berserk?

Though he had only been a medical student for a few months, Morton had absorbed enough of the prevailing medical attitude to predict how Wells's claim would be received. He had also witnessed other demonstrations: Dr. Warren considered it his duty to hear out each and every outrageous claim, in the remote chance that it might benefit medicine. But he was by no means the friendly and helpful fellow that Wells seemed to think he was. To go before Warren with such an absurd claim was foolish. . . . Wells might as well speak to the physics faculty on the subject of a perpetual motion machine, or to demonstrate to engineers that he could fly!

Out of friendship, and in memory of old times, Morton tried to talk reason to Wells, but Wells wouldn't budge from his story. It really worked, Wells kept saying. It really worked!

Morton hesitated. Perhaps someone with a little more authority might be able to pound some sense into Wells's head. While Wells talked on, Morton's mind flipped through the list of imposing people he had met at Harvard. He settled, finally, on Dr. Charles Jackson.

Wells recognized the name, of course, as soon as Morton mentioned it. Anyone who knew anything about science had heard of Dr. Charles Jackson, the chemist and genius. Jackson was the man who had given Samuel Morse the idea for the telegraph machine, during a chance conversation on an ocean liner. Morse denied it, of course, but Jackson was a persuasive man, a gentleman of learning, a man who exuded honesty and integrity. You could believe what you wanted, but everyone knew, and respected, Dr. Jackson. Wells was impressed, despite himself, to find that Morton had such highly placed friends.

Yes, Wells said. He would love to meet Dr. Jackson. Perhaps he would be interested in hearing about nitrous oxide. . . .

Jackson answered the door himself and led them to comfortable seats. Wells watched him, awed. The good chemist was an imposing man, in a professorish way. He had an intelligent-looking face framed with a Quaker's beard, and he wore small eyeglasses perched on his nose. He had thin, stern lips that pursed, thoughtfully, as he listened to Wells tell his story.

When Wells paused for a reaction, Jackson shook his head, sadly. Morton sat silently, watching.

Jackson chose his words carefully, as though to emphasize that each one meant exactly what he meant it to mean, and nothing more or less. He had heard, he said, that ether could make people drunk . . . chemistry students sometimes used it for just that purpose. But then again, alcohol could make people drunk, too, but they woke up fast when the scalpel touched them. The whole idea was just not believable. Pain was a part of existence, and even the world of medicine and surgery had accepted the fact. If Wells went around saying otherwise, he would succeed only in destroying his reputation.

Jackson paused, then added a word of pointed advice. If Wells was wise, he would go to his hotel, pack his bags, and return home to Hartford, his family, and his practice.

Wells was dumbfounded by such scathing criticism from such a respected source. He wanted to scream, "But it works!" and yet . . . the chemist's prediction was a dire one. If he was discredited . . . if a man lost his reputation . . . if Horace lost his reputation he would have nothing left—nothing.

Dejected, he returned to his hotel room to think it through. He sat by a window. The spigot rested in his lap.

But it works!

Perhaps . . .

Drifting, dreaming, the horses' hooves clattering on the pavement below, applause drifting through his mind, bolstering his confidence . . .

Perhaps Jackson was simply wrong.

How could Jackson be wrong? Jackson was . . . well . . . Jackson.

Perhaps Jackson had done nothing wrong; perhaps it was Wells's own fault. Perhaps he hadn't explained it well enough. . . .

Drifting, drifting.

That was it!

He had approached it all wrong!

He had tried to convince Jackson with mere words, whereas deeds were more persuasive.

That solved the problem. Tomorrow's demonstration before the Harvard doctors couldn't help but convince all observers. When he extracted a tooth, painlessly, before their very eyes, they couldn't be skeptical. They couldn't reject the evidence of their own experience, could they? Of course not! It wouldn't be scientific!

He wouldn't go home, no matter what Jackson said.

The resolve was firm, but Jackson's prediction kept edging into his mind, and his heart was racing when he finally pushed into the big Harvard lecture hall, his arms loaded down with equipment.

The amphitheater was full of students, who sat in respectful silence while Warren lectured. Warren didn't appear to notice Wells until the dentist accidentally bumped a wall with one of his boxes. When he did, the surgeon looked over for the first time, an irritated expression on his face. Then he turned his attention back to the class and continued his lecture.

For a moment Wells stood there, half-expecting Warren to interrupt the lecture and introduce him. When it was clear that Warren was going to ignore him, he began setting down the equipment. Remembering the irritation on Warren's face, he tried to be as quiet as possible.

As he stood listening to the lecture's end, Wells's uneasiness grew. In his dreams it had been different. In his dreams he had come to Harvard graciously, a scientific conqueror willing, in the name of humanity, to share his store of knowledge. Back in Hartford, when he had read and reread Warren's letter, the surgeon had seemed warm.

But now, in the reality of the moment, Warren seemed cold and stern. As he talked to the students he delivered his words with a crisp and lofty authority. He never smiled. Wells got the sense that the students were afraid of Warren, and he felt some of that fear himself. He felt, he realized impotently, like a . . . petitioner.

Finally, Warren finished his lecture. He answered a question, ignoring Wells, and then answered another. Finally he paused, examining some papers in front of him,

and his face took on the mildly surprised expression of
someone who had just remembered something minor.

"There's a gentleman here," he said in a formal and patronizing voice, "who pretends he has something which
will destroy pain in surgical operations. He wants to address you. If any of you would like to hear him you may
do so."

Pretends? The blood rushed to Wells's face. *Pretends?*
Pretends?

Warren gathered up his papers, walked into the amphitheater, took a seat in front, drew out a sheaf of papers,
and immediately became absorbed in them.

Wells realized the class was staring at him, and he
reached to pick up his equipment. His fingers seemed
numb and refused to obey him. He dropped something
and then, flustered, dropped something else.

Somehow he got onstage and stood erect before them. A
dental chair, by prearrangement, had been set up on the
stage, and a volunteer with a bad tooth waited in the
wings.

The students had begun to lounge in their seats, and
some of them had their feet up on the chairs in front of
them. One of the students pulled a sandwich out of a bag.
Dr. Warren was still engrossed in the papers. Occasionally
he circled a word or scribbled a note.

Desperately, Wells scanned the audience for a friendly
face. His gaze stopped instead, on Morton. Morton's face
wasn't friendly at all. It wasn't anything. It was blank,
impassive, noncommittal.

Horace groped for words, found them, forgot them, and
cleared his throat instead. Flustered, he dropped the ex-
planatory segment of his plans and turned to introduce the
student who had volunteered for the extraction. The
young man was obviously nervous, and pale with fear.

With Horace's solicitous help, the volunteer settled himself in the chair and opened his mouth wide. Wells bent close to examine the offending tooth, but in his nervousness his elbow brushed across the instrument table and a small tool dropped to the floor. Wells retrieved it but, because his palms were sweaty, it slipped from his grasp and fell again.

There was a chuckle from the audience, then a guffaw that touched off a roar of laughter.

Warren looked up from his papers, fury in his eyes, and the laughter stopped instantly. The silence that followed was absolute.

Ears burning with embarrassment, fingers shaking, Wells dropped still another tool. Somehow he got the nitrous oxide bladder and tube arranged, and handed the volunteer the end of the spigot. The lad sucked on it, as he had been instructed, and seemed to slump down.

Awkwardly, wishing he had brought an assistant, Wells opened the man's mouth, inserted the forceps, grabbed the tooth, rocked, and pulled. As the tooth came free, the patient emitted a low groan that, while not loud, carried well in the chastized silence of the lecture hall.

Horace, accustomed to shrieks, hardly noticed the groan. But the students weren't accustomed to the terrible pain of extractions, and to them the groan signified failure.

As the groan ended and Horace turned, triumphantly, the bloody tooth in the tongs of the forceps, ready at last for the cheers that were his, the lecture hall exploded in derisive laughter.

"*Humbug!*" a voice shouted.

Shocked, Horace turned to the patient, who had recovered and was climbing out of the chair, a grin on his face. Horace bent close to him, to hear his muffled voice over the laughter.

He had felt nothing, nothing at all, the volunteer told Horace.

"Tell them that," Horace begged, pushing the man to the front of the stage. "Quickly! Quickly!"

But with his mouth still bleeding copiously it was difficult for the young man to talk above a whisper, and the students were already on their feet, noisily gathering their papers and talking to one another. Desperately, Wells looked for Morton's face. . . . Morton was a dentist; Morton wouldn't have misinterpreted a groan. . . . But Morton wasn't there. As soon as the laughter erupted, Morton had slipped out of the hall.

Wells stood on the stage for a moment, uncertain, then fled the hall. No one watched him go.

That night in his hotel room, overcome with depression, he sat with the spigot in his lap. The cry of *"Humbug!"* echoed in his skull.

Humbug!

Horace sucked on the tube. It helped.

He hadn't administered enough nitrous, that was all. The patient hadn't been dead drunk. And . . .

And now he was the laughingstock of Boston.

Wave after wave of shame washed through his gas-intoxicated psyche as he relived the debacle again and again, the catcalls ringing anew each time in his ears.

Again he wrapped his lips around the tube and turned the wooden pet cock. The gas had no smell, no smell at all, and the melancholy turned sweet and brought dreams. It hadn't been that bad . . . Morton had been there; *he* was a dentist and *he* had seen; he would explain it all to his fellow students . . . the laughter hadn't happened . . . drifting . . . they had applauded . . . drifting . . . drifting . . . until the bladder was empty.

The next day he returned to Hartford, his wife, his child, and his practice.

Though in his mind the catcalls followed him home, Horace's patients didn't hear them. He naturally used the gas to relieve the pains of his own patients, and the word spread quickly. The callow young men at Harvard could afford to be cynical, but in Hartford people with aching teeth had more open minds. In their desperation, the toothache patients listened to the rumors of a painless dentistry, and while it didn't sound very likely they were willing to try anything, anything at all. They beat a path to his door.

But somehow, to Horace, it wasn't their gratitude that counted. They were from Hartford, not Boston, and they knew nothing of medicine. Boston, and the laughter, followed him everywhere, and no amount of laughing gas could make it go away.

And there was a dullness about him now, a weepiness, a flaccid . . . something that wasn't quite right. He tried more gas, but that didn't help either.

Perhaps, he thought, he was ill. That would explain his failure!

He became increasingly convinced of his illness, and at the urging of his worried and exasperated wife, he went to a physician and was thoroughly examined. The doctor pronounced him healthy.

Healthy? How could he be healthy? For solace, he sat with the spigot in his hands and caressed the problem with his mind.

He walked. Walking helped.

And he worked, in the laboratory, far into the night, trying different things with the gas, breathing it under different circumstances, trying not to remember the laughter and the cry of *"Humbug!"*

In the mornings now, Horace couldn't face his patients. He stayed home, caught in a web of self-hatred and melancholy. He turned away patients. After all, their judgment was meaningless. He had failed in Boston! The hateful guffaws of the medical students followed him into the night, and into his dreams.

Perhaps a new start . . . perhaps . . . He dabbled with an idea for an invention . . . a shower stall . . . one would pour the water into a reservoir in the bottom and then, pumped with one's foot, the water would come out of a spout overhead . . . and he laid the idea aside.

Perhaps an exhibit of some sort. There were a lot of people going around the country with traveling exhibits. Perhaps he could put together an exhibit with birds and stuffed animals . . . or perhaps he should try another invention. . . .

No, he told the patients who came to his door and interrupted his reveries. No, he no longer practiced dentistry, sorry. He was in ill health, you see, and . . .

On April 7, 1845, the following item appeared in the *Hartford Courant:*

DENTAL NOTICE

Having relinquished my professional business for the present, in consequence of ill health, I do with pleasure refer those who have confidence in me to Dr. J. M. Riggs, whose professional qualifications in my opinion are not surpassed by any dentist in the country. This is strong language, but it is said solely for the benefit of my friends who may require any operations on the teeth in my absence.

With the spigot in his lap, Horace fondly remembered the night he had found nitrous oxide, masquerading as "laughing gas" on the lecture circuit. The memory filled him with warm feelings. He envisioned himself on a stage, lecturing on the subject of naturalism. The audience, he was certain, wouldn't laugh. . . .

Two months later an advertisement appeared.

WELLS PANORAMA OF NATURE

H. Wells will give a series of Entertain-
ments, embracing the subject of Natural
History, at the City Hall, commencing this
evening, Monday, June 2. Major Ham-
ilton's Brass Band will be in attendance.
Single tickets 25 cents. Tickets admitting a
Lady and a Gentleman, 37½ cents. Children under 12 years of age at half price.
Doors open at 7:30, commence at 8 o'clock.

Horace's family and friends couldn't comprehend why
he was abandoning dentistry. Hadn't he the key to painless dentistry in his grasp? Wasn't that the key to wealth
and prestige?

At least, they urged him, at least . . . for the good of
your wife and child, if nothing else . . . at least patent the
laughing gas procedure!

Wells listened to their advice, thought about it, and
prayed for guidance, but his answer was negative. He explained as patiently as he knew how that he couldn't, in
good Christian conscience, apply for a patent. A patent
might serve to restrict the use of nitrous, and the technique was simply too important, and offered too much
benefit to suffering humanity, to be restricted.

The gas should in fact be free, free as the air, for all
who were or ever would be in agony. As for his wife and
children, he would dutifully provide for them himself. He
was planning a lecture, he explained. . . .

Meanwhile, in Boston, Morton couldn't shake the image of
Wells pulling a tooth painlessly, and it *had* been painless,
no matter what the students thought. Morton had the
good sense to keep his mouth shut about it—he had no
desire to be hooted down, as Wells had been—but all the
same, he thought about it.

On the one hand, Wells was no humbug. The patient should have been screaming and begging for mercy, not groaning. A groan was nothing. On the other hand Wells shouldn't have allowed the groan to occur. He should have known the procedure backward and forward before attempting to demonstrate it at Harvard. Wells wasn't a humbug, but he was certainly an incautious and sloppy fool. He had been surprised by the groan, and therein lay his fatal error.

If he, Morton, were to offer such a demonstration, he wouldn't make any mistakes at all. He would be perfectly prepared and there would be no surprises.

For the moment Morton was engrossed in his studies, but that summer, in the heat of July, he found time to travel to Hartford and visit his old teacher. He told Horace that he believed him, even if nobody else did, and that he would like to do some experimentation on his own.

Horace greeted his onetime student and partner with open arms, but when Morton asked for some nitrous oxide to take back to Boston, the bitterness welled up. Where had Morton been in the hour of need? Why hadn't he stayed in the amphitheater, in support of his friend?

No, Wells refused to give him any gas. If Morton wanted gas, why didn't he approach his chemist friend, the self-proclaimed inventor of the telegraph, what's-his-name, Dr. Jackson?

Thus rebuffed, Morton withdrew as politely as he could and returned home. And he did pay a call on Jackson.

Jackson discussed the matter with Morton, but he was skittish about getting involved. It seemed to him that a scientist like himself could destroy his reputation with a fraudulent-sounding idea like painless surgery. After all, remember Wells. Hadn't he ruined himself in a single hour?

No, Jackson wasn't about to get involved, but, he said, if Morton was really going to be so foolish as to pursue the matter he should at least reject the idea of using a gas. Try ether, instead. Gas wouldn't work. Jackson was certain of that. And besides, ether was easy to get.

Morton hadn't the time at the moment to do any research, but when the term ended he purchased a bottle of ether to take with him to his family's country home in West Needham. That summer, while Wells tinkered with stuffed birds and worked on designing a newfangled bathing device back in Hartford, Morton searched for a guinea pig upon which to test the stupor-producing qualities of ether.

His attention focused on Nig, the family's cocker spaniel. Nig looked back at him trustingly and wagged his tail.

"C'mon, Nig," said Morton, and he led the dog downstairs to the basement.

Morton put some cotton in a saucer and poured some ether on it. He beckoned to Nig and, when the dog responded, he grabbed it and held its muzzle above the saucer. Nig resisted at first, but the struggles quickly became feeble, then stopped altogether. Finally Morton released his grip.

Nig crumpled to the basement floor, unconscious.

For a moment Morton sat and looked at the inert animal, satisfied. A minute passed, then two, then three.

Slowly, Morton's sense of accomplishment turned to alarm. He nudged the animal and got no response. He shook it violently, still to no avail.

He waited.

What would he tell his wife, Elizabeth? The thought filled him with dread.

Did the dog move?

"Nig?"

A front leg twitched, then a back one. Nig snorted and moved his head.

Morton breathed a sigh of relief. That settled the question of what to say to Elizabeth. He would say nothing.

But Morton wasn't adept at clandestine experimentation, and the secrecy was short-lived. The next day, when
Elizabeth noticed that the goldfish bowl was empty, her
intuition led her immediately to her husband's study. Sure
enough, the goldfish were lying, obviously dead, on a
workbench.

Defensively, Morton maintained that he'd done no
harm. To demonstrate, he put the fish back into the bowl
and in a few moments they started swimming around. As
Elizabeth acidly pointed out, they did seem a little slug-
gish . . . but they were alive, nonetheless. Soon they
would be as good as new.

The prolonged exchange that followed was, as they say,
quite memorable. Before it was over a humbled Morton
had confessed all, including his experiments on Nig. He
wouldn't use the dog again, he promised. Or the goldfish.
Or any other pets. By the time Elizabeth was finished he
was limited to crawly things from the garden and fish
from the pond.

For a while he was content with minnows, worms, and
beetles. But it was mammals that counted.

He looked at Nig speculatively, and Nig, wiser now,
edged away.

That left Morton very little choice. He poured ether
into the waiting saucer, capped the bottle, set it aside, and
leaned over the saucer.

In what seemed like an instant, but had probably been
much longer, it was all over. He was slumped over the
table, his head resting on its side. He sat up, a little
groggy, and gave his head time to clear. When it did he
mentally checked himself over. He was fine. Everything
was normal. Well, not exactly normal. "Exhilarated" was a
better word. Fantasies of fame and money swirled through
his brain.

He promised himself he would go slowly, plan carefully, and leave no room for surprises.

In the meantime, back in Hartford, Wells had drifted
away from the exhibition project and gone back to experimenting with nitrous. He sat at his desk, pencil and pad in
front of him, for hours, spigot in hand, thinking, drifting,
dreaming . . . measuring. He wouldn't take the gas for
himself, only for science. . . .

If only he had performed the demonstration better. If
only the groan hadn't occurred. If only he knew how
much gas exactly it took to anesthetize a patient. If only he
knew, and could predict, the different tolerances of different patients. If only, if only, if only.

He sat, thinking, breathing the gas, dreaming, drifting,
drifting, inhaling deeply . . .

Finally, by autumn, the laughter and catcalls had receded far enough for him to recognize impending bank-
ruptcy. Perhaps his relatives were correct. He couldn't
patent nitrous . . . that would be immoral. But he could
go back into practice.

He placed an ad in the *Courant*, and the response impressed everyone but him. Soon he was standing for hours
in his bloody apron, administering the gas, pulling the
tooth, then stepping back while that patient left, looking
surprised, and another, looking terrified, took his place. In
the months that followed he painlessly extracted teeth
from a steady stream of mouths, some of which belonged
to extremely influential people—including an Episcopalian
bishop and two of his daughters.

And so as 1845 ended and the spring and summer of
1846 passed, Wells's existence faded into the routine of
work. The stuffed animals gathered dust and his new patent for a foot-pump shower stall lay ignored. He was a
success, suddenly, by any definition but his own.

The laughter and catcalls didn't surge through his head

as often now, but he was subject to an ever increasing melancholia. Money didn't help. Elizabeth didn't help. Nothing seemed to help . . . nothing but the experiments. When he sat with the spigot in his lap the blue ache left his brain and he could dream again, as he had before, of applause. The experiments were all that kept him going.

In Boston, meanwhile, a prominent citizen named Eben Frost developed a terrible toothache that wouldn't go away. He suffered it for a few days but, instead of getting better, it got worse. He faced the terrible decision. Yes, he would have to go to a dentist. The thought made his heart pound in terror, his hands turn clammy and cold. He clenched and unclenched them.

Which dentist?

He knew a man . . . who . . . his name was . . . oh . . . Morton. Morton was a doctor, but he had once been a dentist, and he was known for his distaste for a patient's pain. . . . Perhaps he could arrange for a hypnotist. Perhaps a hypnotist . . .

Morton at the time was in his office, discussing other matters with a Dr. Hayden. When Frost arrived, obviously in misery, Morton motioned him into the office and he and Dr. Hayden listened to his plea.

As Frost talked, Morton recognized his opportunity. Unlike Wells, he was ready. He had been patient and waited. Now providence had provided his opportunity.

A hypnotist? Morton snorted. Frauds and fakers, every one! But, Morton said, he had something better. It was called ether.

Morton assured Frost that he had tried the procedure on animals and even on himself, and that it was perfectly safe. First, he said, taking a bottle of ether, I sprinkle a little on my handkerchief, and then . . .

He placed the handkerchief over Frost's nose. Frost struggled momentarily, then lost consciousness. Morton reached for the forceps, closed them around the tooth, rocked, and yanked. The only sound was the clink of the tooth hitting the floor. Morton, in his excitement, had let it drop.

The two doctors stared at it, Hayden with surprise and Morton with glee. Soon Frost recovered and was told his ordeal was over . . . and he had slept through it. Then he, too, stared at amazement at the tooth.

Morton waited until Frost had stopped bleeding and then asked both men to follow him.

Where?

To the editorial offices of the *Boston Daily Journal*, where else?

The next day's newspaper heralded the birth of painless dentistry and described the use of ether by Dr. William Morton.

It was one thing to convince the public, of course, and quite another to win over the doctors. Morton knew his next step was a giant one. He made an appointment to see Dr. John Collins Warren, the medical school surgeon who had presided over Wells's humiliation.

Warren, who had seen Morton among the medical students, offered him a chair. Morton sat on the edge of it while he explained what he wanted to do.

Warren watched the young man over the top rim of his eyeglasses. Warren had had the impression Morton was a smart fellow. Impressions, of course, could be grossly deceptive.

Over the years Warren had suffered through countless demonstrations prepared by idiots, numbskulls, and frauds. He reckoned that he owed his own student, however balmy, at least as much attention as he awarded, say, some bumpkin dentist from Hartford. He had squandered over an hour of his time on that one, when was it? A year ago? Two?

Warren's mind sorted through its mental file of current

patients and settled on a young man with a tumor in his neck. The lad had been dreading the operation and so, in truth, had the surgeon. The agony was going to be incredible. If nothing else, Morton's experiment might give the patient some hope, something to help keep up his courage until the moment arrived. That could be useful. Morton certainly couldn't do anything about the pain, but he might help alleviate its anticipation.

Morton left the office elated. He knew Warren didn't expect him to succeed, but that was all to the good. He would be that much more impressed when the boy felt no pain.

Morton stopped.

If it worked, might he be accused of risking the patient's life?

Morton himself knew for certain it was safe, but he had consulted nobody on the subject. Once the thought occurred to him, it worried him. It was the one thing he hadn't thought of, and it shook his confidence.

He altered his course, heading now for Dr. Jackson's office. Jackson would certainly certify that ether was safe. After all, he had recommended it in the first place, hadn't he?

The logic was so impeccable that Morton was doubly surprised when Jackson refused, and accused Morton of being on a fool's errand. It would turn out badly in the end, the chemist predicted. He, Jackson, wasn't about to have his good name associated with any such harebrained scheme.

Morton left Jackson's apartment and started walking home. By the time he arrived, he had decided to shrug off Jackson's attitude and go ahead with the experiment. Of course it was safe! All ether did, or nitrous oxide either, for that matter, was put you to sleep. Where was the danger in that?

He didn't have a certification of safety, but in all other

respects he was prepared. Unlike Wells, he knew the inner
workings of the Boston medical world, and he knew how
to discreetly attract interest. A word here and a word
there and, on October 16, 1846, as the terrified boy was
wheeled into the operating theater, the place was packed
with students and doctors, all craning their necks to see.
Whatever else happened, Morton wouldn't be ignored.

Morton produced a funnel with an ether-soaked piece of
cotton in it and placed the small end in the patient's
mouth. Obeying Morton's instructions, the boy took a
deep breath, gagged slightly, and desperately took another
and then another. Soon his breathing became shallow and
Morton stepped back.

"Your patient is ready," he said to Warren.

Working quickly, as he was accustomed to doing, Warren sliced into the patient's neck, expecting to hear a
scream. When there was no scream he hesitated, looking
up at Morton.

There were still no screams.

Morton nodded politely and smiled.

Without saying a word, Warren directed his attention
back to the job at hand. Blood flowed, and was staunched
with clips. Soon the tumor lay, a lump of flesh, in a pan.
The incision was stitched up.

Warren stepped back.

"Gentlemen," he announced in an incredulous voice,
"gentlemen . . . *this is not humbug!*"

All the correct people had seen the feat, and the word
spread rapidly. The name Morton reverberated through
the American medical world and crossed to Europe, in
dozens of letters, on the next packet. A journal article appeared, and Morton was suddenly much in demand as a
medical school lecturer.

But the success was not without encumbrances. Within
a month of the demonstration he got a bill from Dr. Jack-

son. He read it, puzzled. The chemist demanded five hundred dollars for "professional advice" leading to the invention of the new ether procedure.

Morton stared at the bill in disbelief. Was this the same Jackson who wouldn't even certify that ether was safe, lest he sully his precious reputation?

And if Dr. Jackson's claim surprised him, he was astonished by the erratic behavior of his old teacher and friend—he had thought—from back in Hartford. Morton had written Wells a letter, telling him that his dream of painless dentistry and surgery as well had been achieved. He even suggested that, once a patent was obtained, Horace might want to serve as his agent.

He had expected congratulations. Instead he had gotten back an almost incoherent letter from Wells saying, in effect, *stop everything*. A few days later the distraught dentist was in Morton's office, demanding to see ether used.

Morton arranged for him to see an operation, and he did. He didn't say a word until the procedure was over, and then he confronted Morton. There was no substantial difference, he said, between Morton's use of ether and Wells's earlier use of nitrous oxide. It was all the same, in principle. The invention, Horace said, wasn't Morton's to patent. It belonged, instead, to Wells.

Morton listened to the argument, but he refused to rise to the bait. He willingly acknowledged his debt to Wells and even offered, in fairness, to cut him in on the profits—if there were any. But it was only fair that he, Morton, get the credit. After all, Wells's demonstration had failed, hadn't it? Morton's had succeeded, hadn't it? Fair was fair.

Wells stared at his old student, his onetime friend who had now stolen his invention. In a daze, Wells turned and walked away, not hearing Morton's halfhearted attempts to call him back.

Morton was sorrier about Wells, because of the onetime

friendship, but Jackson was the better-equipped pre-
tender. Already he was going around telling anyone who
would listen that it was all his idea, that he had been experimenting with ether for half a decade. Hearing reports
of these claims, Morton decided he was beginning to understand how Samuel Morse felt.

Morton himself had made it worse by attempting to buy
Jackson off. Morton replied to the bill with an offer to pay
a 10 percent royalty, figuring that would satisfy the chemist. But it was the wrong move. Jackson now pointed to
the offer as a tacit admission that it had been his idea all
along.

Partly to rebut this contention, and also to demonstrate
that he, Morton, was actively at work on the project, he
began publishing a weekly circular called *Letheon*, in which
he reported the results of his continuing ether trials both
in the laboratory and in the operating theater.

Back in Hartford, Wells complained bitterly to his wife
and friends that Morton had stolen his idea, but he was
impotent to do anything about it. He was sad, but not
surprised, when a patent was issued in 1846 for a substance that was described only as Letheon. Letheon, Wells
assumed, was a fancy name for the ether that could be
purchased in any pharmacy.

Wells read in the *Boston Evening Transcript* that the patent applied to a means "whereby pain may be prevented in
dental and surgical operations." The paper said that the
patent had been issued jointly to Morton and Jackson.
Wells wasn't sure what Jackson had to do with it. The
credit by all rights should be his, Horace's!

He watched in despair from the sidelines as the medical
and popular press beat the drums for Letheon. The story
of Morton's demonstration had traveled around the world,
and one famous surgeon after another confirmed, in letters
to journals, the amazing qualities of Letheon. Speculation
grew that, with a sense-deadening chemical, surgeons

might actually be able to cut into the abdomen without killing the patient. In England, Dr. James Young Simpson heard about ether and began a search for something even better, a search that would lead eventually to the use of chloroform.

There was a reaction, as well, from established interests. Dentists who didn't have licenses from Morton to use Letheon established a "Committee of Vigilance" as a propaganda clearinghouse. The committee released reports charging that patients had died under ether, or had been plagued for weeks afterward by melancholia. A rumor, given credence by the committee, said that the substance made young virgins licentious. When they woke up, they remembered nothing. Hearing this charge, mothers spent a speculative moment thinking about daughters who had taken ether.

Some of the articles mentioned Morton and others referred to Jackson, while a few credited both. Horace's name never appeared, but he followed the events avidly. In his office, his desk was soon piled high with journal articles, clippings, and letters.

Wells learned that Jackson had written a secret letter to France in an attempt to establish his claim with the scientific societies in Paris, at that time the most prestigious in the Western world. In response, Morton sent a representative to argue his claims before the learned societies of Europe and, at the same time, petitioned Congress to give him an award for the discovery of anesthesia. Jackson lobbied Congress in his own behalf, effectively bogging down Morton's cause in controversy.

Story after story appeared in the newspapers and was clipped out and added to the jumbled pile on Wells's desk in Hartford. Finally, two weeks before Christmas of 1846, Horace poured out his version of the story in a letter to the local *Courant*.

He told about his ill-fated experiment in Boston, and

acknowledged that he had removed the nitrous oxide too soon. But, he claimed, the patient had testified to feeling no pain. Consequently, regardless of the audience reaction, the experiment had been successful and established his priority with the discovery. He hoped, he said, that the *Courant*'s readers would consider the matter impartially and make up their own minds about who deserved credit.

He read the letter, when it appeared, over and over. The nitrous oxide spigot in his lap made the letter appear devastating. It should establish his claim, he told himself, once and for all.

Reaching for pen and paper, he composed a letter to Morton in which he asserted that he had the power to invalidate the patent "by a word."

Yet, Wells wrote, it wasn't money that drove him and, as long as he and Morton remained on good terms, he would do no such thing. But he would, he vowed, achieve the public recognition that was due him.

Wells posted the letter and waited . . . for what? Nothing, really, had changed. While Morton and Jackson told their stories to select scientific audiences, he was reduced to pouring out his heart to the local newspaper! He had waited long enough. It was time to act.

Turning over his practice to another dentist, Wells booked passage to Europe. In Paris, he was sure, an impartial academy would believe him. He had little money, but he was certain he could pay for the trip by purchasing engravings on the Continent and bringing them home to sell at a profit.

Jackson, in the meantime, had begun to contradict himself and resort to name-calling. He claimed to have discovered the anesthetic properties of ether in 1842, but hadn't pursued the matter because ether was known to be poisonous. He also labeled Morton a quack and an ignoramus.

Why then, he was eventually asked, did he suggest to a quack and an ignoramus—Morton—that he use ether on his patients?

Jackson was caught short for a moment, but only a moment. Relying on his audience's ignorance and short memory, he blithely replied that ether was known to be harmless, and therefore could be handled even by a quack and an ignoramus. Such answers served to confuse the audience and leave his critics sputtering in impotent outrage.

In Paris, in the meantime, Wells disembarked to discover, to his horror, that the scientific societies had, on the basis of Jackson's letter, already given the chemist presumptive credit for the discovery of anesthesia. The Paris Medical Institute had even granted a 2,500-franc award to Jackson and, as a peace-keeping afterthought, voted the same sum to Morton for his work in the discovery's application.

And who, the French scientists asked politely, was Horace Wells? A dentist? From Hartford? And where, please, is Hartford? . . .

Horace hadn't been able to bring nitrous oxide to Europe. The equipment was too bulky and didn't travel well. Fortunately he had switched to ether, which was carried in jars and, when sniffed correctly, also banished the melancholia that, abetted by a callous world, was never far away from him. With ether he could continue to dream, to face each day, to explain again and again and again that the credit should be his.

The story fell mostly on skeptical ears, but Wells found an immediate ally in an American dentist working in Paris, Dr. C. S. Brewster. For years Brewster had endured the superior attitude of Europeans toward "backward Yankees," and was now overjoyed with the turn of events. The discovery of anesthesia had become the talk of the Parisian cafés, and Brewster was only too pleased to escort another Important American Scientist around town.

Largely as a result of Brewster's efforts, Wells was allowed to appear before the Academy of Sciences, the Academy of Medicine, and the Parisian Medical Society.

He recounted each time how he had gone to Colton's lecture in 1844, and how the next day he had used Colton's laughing gas—nitrous oxide—to have one of his own teeth extracted painlessly. He told of his experiments on himself, of his painless treatment of his patients, and of his disastrous demonstration in Boston. He tried to keep his voice from quavering with anger as he charged that neither Jackson nor Morton had supported him at the time, but that later each had announced the discovery of anesthesia without mentioning the name Horace Wells or acknowledging his germinal contribution.

It was true, Wells explained, that Morton had been the first to use ether for anesthesia. Others were experimenting with different substances, and new gases and vaporous liquids would undoubtedly be found. But wasn't it the discovery of the principle that should receive the most credit?

After each presentation Brewster reported to him that the mood was favorable, but that the scientists continued to have misgivings. The presentations were just words, after all. Where was the proof that Wells had been first?

Brewster suggested that Wells return home quickly, compile the statements and affidavits necessary to prove his claim, and send them by packet to Paris. Brewster promised that he would make certain the material got into the hands of the right people.

Wells concurred, stopping only long enough to present his version of the story to the Royal Society of Medicine in London. From there, his supply of ether replenished in England, he sailed to Boston.

Horace arrived home to find that the controversy over the discovery of anesthesia had been joined by yet another contender. A country doctor from the South, Crawford

Long, claimed to have used ether for years but to have neglected to report it.

Though Long was getting a hearing, Wells rejected the claim out of hand. Even if the story was true, what was the significance of a discovery if it went unreported? If Long knew a way of alleviating pain, why did he deny it to a suffering world?

Before returning home to Hartford to put together a package for the French societies, Wells stopped in Boston to meet with representatives of Morton and Jackson. But there was no room for negotiation. Wells angrily proclaimed that he wanted no money . . . but the credit was his and, with the help of God, he would see justice done.

At home, Wells worked singlemindedly to document his claims. Samuel Cooley, the pharmacist whose bruised shin had begun it all, signed a statement that he had witnessed Riggs pulling Wells's tooth in 1844. Riggs added his own sworn statement. Dozens of patients added affidavits that their teeth had been pulled painlessly, long before Morton had made any claim. The package of documents was given special weight because it included an affidavit from the Episcopalian bishop.

Wells put the evidence in the mail in March, and went home to a lonely house and a cold supper. Elizabeth had taken their son and moved in with her parents.

Stubbornly, Horace clung to his dream of recognition. Pain . . . what was pain?

It was the screeching agony of a tooth pulling free of the jaw, the horrible torment of the surgeon's knife. But it was also a quiet and desperate thing that had no blood at all, that moved through the mind with ghosts of past wrongs, of mistakes, of guilts, of melancholia that swept away happiness with waves of misery, slow, killing . . .

There were two kinds of pain, and nitrous helped them both. So did ether.

Horace bent over his desk, inhaling deeply, forgetting

to eat, thinking, hating, sailing into a sea of drugged bitterness, abandoning himself to the drug psychosis.

Spring came and the redbud bloomed. Petunias appeared in the flowerboxes of Hartford. Summer passed, almost unremembered, in the bloodless pain. Then the weather cooled and frost painted the trees. There was no word from Paris. Newspaper articles and rumors from Boston told Wells of the raging battle between Morton and Jackson.

Wells struggled to pull himself from his emotional morass. He knew he must do something, take some action to stop the confusing passage of months.

Perhaps a change of place, a city more befitting his importance, perhaps Boston . . . no. Not Boston. The cry of *"humbug!"* echoed in his mind. Not Boston. Certainly not Boston, but a big city, a city that would appreciate . . .

Horace put the nitrous tube in his mouth and breathed deeply, stilling the cacophony of derisive catcalls. Autumn passed into winter and snow covered Connecticut. Word came from Europe of the discovery of still another anesthetizing chemical, chloroform.

Horace obtained some and sampled it. He was impressed. As he told anyone who would listen, it was far better than Morton's ether.

It, too, served to banish the laughter, to make the future seem bright, the present more tolerable. It helped him forget that the world was full of enemies, enemies everywhere, squabbling over the fruits of his labor, his lifework . . .

New York, then. In New York he could start over. . . .

On January 7, 1848, an advertisement appeared in the *New York Herald* announcing the arrival of Dr. Horace Wells, the noted surgeon-dentist, "the discoverer of ether and various stimulating gases used in annulling pain, now . . . willing to attend to those who might require his personal services."

But in New York, bereft of family, friends, and dreams, his mind slipped its last moorings and foundered in a sea of confusion and pain.

As he waited for patients, Horace discovered that alcohol by mouth and chloroform vapors by lungs combined to produce a particularly intoxicating effect . . . he could write it down later . . . laughter . . . Christmas . . . what year? . . . Elizabeth . . . Elizabeth? . . . where were Elizabeth and the child? . . . enemies everywhere . . . evil, evil was everywhere . . . friends . . . friends were few and precious . . .

He craved friends and he found one on the street.

The friend was a young man who had chatted with Horace in the park, and who was easily enticed back to the office for further conversation. The man was a good listener and Horace, his mind clouded with nitrous oxide, ether, chloroform, and alcohol in combination, poured out the whole, hateful story.

His young friend, in return, recounted his own troubles. Why, only the other day he had been assaulted on Broadway by some low woman, some prostitute. He had rejected her offer with more curtness than she had perhaps expected, and the wretch had responded by throwing some drops of acid on him. The acid had ruined his coat and the man was furious.

Sharing one another's paranoia and indignation, the two talked of "driving all the bad girls off Broadway."

Horace had some acid, he said. Sulfuric acid. It was in a glass bottle with a cork in it, and the cork could be altered to allow just a few drops to escape.

The man put the bottle in the pocket of an old coat, and he and Horace returned to Broadway. Soon the girl was spotted. Horace's friend ran up to her, sprinkled several drops of acid on her coat, and then ran.

Later, back in his office, Horace put the acid bottle back on the shelf and sat down to think about it all, a bottle of chloroform and a bottle of alcohol before him. As he sat and drank and breathed the fumes, the incident of the prostitute grew larger and more significant in his drug-twisted mind.

It seemed to Horace that his friend's experience, getting his coat ruined with acid, was very representative of life. A man worked hard, did the moral thing, achieved something . . . and then some horrid, evil person stepped out of the shadows and attacked him.

Horace was glad his friend had had his revenge. Perhaps . . . perhaps in that way, by attacking evil directly, it could be defeated. Perhaps all the bad girls could be driven off Broadway entirely, forced back into the narrow side streets. . . .

The laughter roared in his mind, and he silenced it with alcohol and chloroform. A day passed. Two. He treated patients, pulled teeth, put the money in his cashbox.

The chloroform and alcohol helped. Together, he told himself, they allowed him to think more clearly, to see and identify the evil around him. The chemicals allowed him to understand that the evil had to stop. It had to stop somewhere. There had to be justice, retribution. . . .

The melancholia rose in his mind. . . . Elizabeth? . . . He breathed deeply, inhaling the chloroform again and again until he slumped sideways. He awoke.

He didn't know what time it was.

There was evil, evil all around, evil on the streets.

Alarmed, he grabbed the bottle of sulfuric acid and dashed outside to confront it. He stopped on the street and looked both ways, hesitating.

It was cold. There were two women on the corner, evil women; he could tell by their dress, by their very presence on the corner. . . .

He lunged at them, screaming out his hatred and frustration, drops of acid flying. The women shrieked, covering their faces.

Broadway.

Which way was Broadway? The evil was on Broadway. . . .

Evil. Evil everywhere. Injustice everywhere. They were after him. There was a loud whistle. The streets were in the hands of painted women and felons, and the police were in their pay. He ran.

A firm hand grasped his right shoulder, spinning him around. Someone took him from behind, and a blue-uniformed arm wrapped itself around his neck. He struggled, without success.

He felt the professional pat of hands on his coat and trousers, searching for weapons. Suddenly, Horace stopped fighting.

A young officer stood before Horace, giving him a long and appraising look, noting the chloroform-crazed eyes and unkempt appearance. The officer called for manacles.

As Horace sat on the sidewalk waiting for the paddy wagon and the long, lurching ride to the station beside common criminals, his mind ceased to process new information. He saw the petty thieves who sat beside him, heard the clop of the horses' hooves on the cobblestones, heard—and obeyed—the officer's command to climb down and line up along the wall. He smelled the icy stench of the Tombs in winter. Someone, a judge, asked him who he was, and Horace tried to explain.

After he told them his identity they treated him with more respect. The assault charges weren't dismissed, but they put him in a private cell.

He sat, alone, with no alcohol or chloroform, defenseless against the melancholia. It was cold in the Tombs, but he sweated profusely nonetheless, and his hands shook without explanation. The laughter echoed in his head.

Chloroform would help, but he didn't have any. Perhaps . . . He asked the jailer if he could go home and get some things . . . some toilet articles. The jailer agreed.

A policeman took him to his apartment and waited by the door while Horace packed a few belongings into a traveling case. A suit. Some socks. Underwear. A hairbrush . . . He moved into the bathroom. The policeman didn't follow. The chloroform bottle quickly disappeared into the suitcase.

He needed some other things, too. A toothbrush. A wash cloth. Soap . . .

His mind froze as his eyes met themselves, reflected in the mirror. He stopped, staring.

He hardly recognized the face that gazed back at him. It did look crazed, crazed and old . . . prematurely old, the face of a beggar in the streets, of a drunkard in the alley, a face to laugh at . . . laugh at . . . laugh at . . . laugh at . . .

He looked away, and his eyes rested on his straight razor. He picked it up and examined it, almost with surprise. It was his razor, he knew that, but it was as though he had never seen it before.

Slowly, he folded the handle over the blade's edge and put it, along with a cup of dried-up shaving soap, into his bag. Then he snapped the bag closed and returned to the waiting policeman.

Horace's mind was calm now, and steady. The laughter was still there but it seemed distant, almost beyond hearing. He sat back in the carriage seat, watched the buildings glide by beyond the glass, and chatted about the weather with the officer beside him.

His was a special cell, for gentlemen who got into trouble. There was a desk in it, and as the afternoon and evening passed he sat at it and wrote.

"Gentlemen," he wrote to the editors of the *Journal of Commerce*, "I wish, through the medium of this journal, to make a plain statement respecting the unhappy circumstances in which I am at present placed. . . ."

He stopped, listening for the footfall of a guard. He heard nothing. It was late and the Tombs was silent. Stealthily, Horace removed the bottle of chloroform and held it under his nose for a moment.

". . . My name is before the public as a miscreant, guilty of a most despicable act, that of wantonly destroying the property of those girls of the town who nightly promenade Broadway. . . ."

The hour passed. Far away, a churchbell chimed. The words came slowly, delivered in humility and pain.

". . . To explain . . . I had been in the constant practice of inhaling chloroform for the exhilarating effect. . . . I have done this one act in a moment of delirium. . . . My dear wife and child, oh, may God protect them! I cannot proceed, my hand is too unsteady. . . . My brain is on fire. . . .

"Great God! has it come to this. . . . If I was to go free tomorrow I could not live and be called a villain. God knows I am not one. Oh, my dear mother, brother and sister, what can I say to you. . . . Oh! what misery I shall bring upon all my relatives. . . . My dear wife and child, whom I leave destitute of the means of support . . . Were I to live on I would become a maniac. . . . I feel that I am fast becoming a deranged man. . . . I cannot live and keep my reason. . . ."

He signed the letter, lay down on his bed, inhaled the chloroform, opened the razor, hesitated, put the razor down, and sat up. Not yet.

He returned to the desk to add a note to the editors, begging them to be kind to Elizabeth.

He lay down again, got up, and added a note to Elizabeth herself. Again he lay down, prepared himself, hesitated, rose, and returned to his desk. This time, in the interest of probate, he listed the items to be included in his estate, including his dentist's chair, sixteen yards of carpet on the floor, some sea shells, assorted forceps, and a dollar's worth of gold.

He lay back down on the bed and held his nose over the chloroform bottle for a long time. He knew precisely the dose he needed.

Just before he passed out he forced the razor deep into his thigh. The femoral artery pumped a torrent of blood onto the sheets. Then he lay in liquid red warmth, drifting, dreaming, suffering no more, true anesthesia finally achieved.

A few days after Horace's death, an urgent letter arrived on a packet from France. The letter went first to Hartford, but the dentist had gone, it was said, to New York. So the letter went to New York, by fast carriage, but in New York it was learned that the addressee was recently deceased. The letter was readdressed to the next of kin and sent back to Hartford, where it was given to Mrs. Elizabeth Wells.

She looked at the envelope, puzzled. The return address was that of a Dr. C. S. Brewster. Who was Dr. C. S. Brewster? She hesitated a moment, then ripped the seal open.

History would show that Dr. Crawford Long had indeed discovered anesthesia first but, because he was afraid his puritanical peer group would disown him, kept the discovery secret. He would be judged, for all time, the coward who kept pain alive.

Dr. Morton would be credited with introducing anesthesia into surgery, but his life would be ruined by Jackson, who would dog him to his death and beyond with legal claims.

As for Dr. Jackson, he would eventually be recognized as the fraud and con artist he was. He would ultimately be found, screaming claims and accusations, on Morton's grave. He would be taken to an asylum, where he would eventually die.

The letter from France contained the first news that the reappraisal was taking place. In a judgment that history would follow, the Parisian Medical Society had decided that it was Horace Wells who had discovered anesthesia. While nitrous oxide had already given way to ether, and that would one day be superseded by modern anesthetics like halothane, the credit belonged to Wells, and Wells alone.

But the ultimate irony of the story wouldn't be understood for a century, and then only vaguely. The chemicals that deadened physical pain did so by acting directly on the brain where, the puritans knew instinctively, every pain is counterbalanced by pleasure and every pleasure by pain. Horace Wells banished physical pain and opened the way for modern surgery, but in doing so he also discovered an escape from the grinding ache of reality. That, in turn, laid the foundation for a new era of psychosis, addiction, anguish, and suicide.

History records him as the discoverer of anesthesia, and as its first victim.

THE RIDDLE OF THE RÍMAC VALLEY

Along the Pacific edge of South America, where the continent grinds relentlessly over the seabed and the living stone buckles skyward, the Andes rise in three distinct ranges. Beneath their ice-carved peaks the capital city of Lima, Peru, stands by the tropical sea.

From this city Spanish viceroys once ruled the ancient Inca empire, but by the middle 1800s their palaces were occupied by aristocrats who called themselves Peruvian but who reigned largely by right of their Spanish blood.

The wealth of the country came from the high interior, from the Andes, from the eternal labor of the Indian, from the stone itself, from places like Cerro de Pasco.

There, on the high arid plateau between the first two lines of peaks, Indians wriggled through deep burrows, scratching for silver and copper. The rock, collected in small baskets, was carried to the surface and smelted in crude furnaces; then the ingots were loaded on llamas for the trip to the seaport below.

In Lima the metals were sold and the pack animals loaded with luxuries for the return trip. There were knives of good steel, material woven in Europe, furniture of German oak, oils from Pacific whales, spices, books—almost all destined for the families of the mixed-blood mine su-

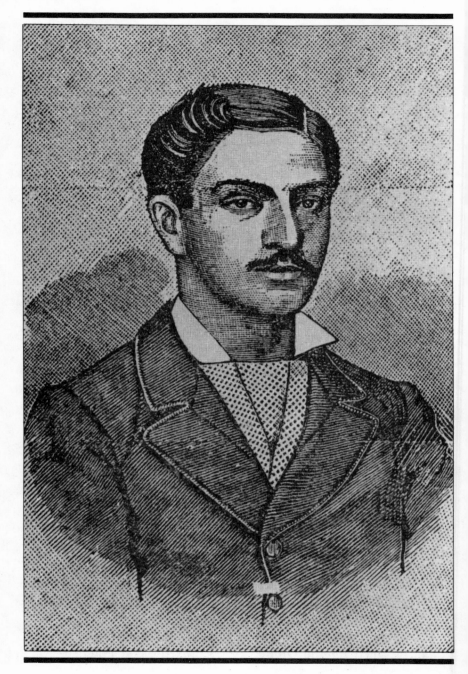

DANIEL A. CARRIÓN

Courtesy Dr. José Whittembury

pervisors, priests, doctors, and lawyers who composed the aristocracy of the high tableland.

Today the trip from Lima to Cerro de Pasco is measured at perhaps 175 miles, but in 1858, the year Daniel Carrión was born in the land of the condor, it was reckoned in time. Six days.

The first twenty-three miles from Lima to Chosica were relatively easy, and merchandise was loaded on the strong backs of mules. But then, when the incline grew more pronounced, the loads were transferred to llamas. The llamas moved more slowly than the mules and carried a far smaller load, but the mules couldn't survive the heights to come.

All the way the trail followed the Rímac River, a green and silver torrent that dropped more than twenty thousand feet in just sixty miles. Beyond San Bartolomé the traveler climbed into a canyon of beauty and horror.

Where the river cut into the Andean uplift, sheets of rock rose vertically above the powerful current. A deafening roar filled the canyon, echoing from rock face to rock face, and in such places the trail was no more than a groove cut in the cliff.

The dainty feet of the llamas struck within inches of the precipice, but men were more likely than animals to tumble screaming into the abyss. Sometimes ice storms blew down without warning from the nearby peaks, and handholds were carved into the rock.

The Rímac Valley, or as much of it as was habitable, was populated by a quiet Indian people who suffered stoically at the hands of a local demon. They said the creature spent its days in a hole, emerging to hunt at night. Invisible, it revealed its presence only through the swarm of tiny sand flies that followed it wherever it went. It grabbed its prey in many-fingered hands, and where each transparent fingertip touched skin, a hideous and painful red wart would grow.

If the victim had been born in the valley, the demon would usually set him loose to develop the warts and serve as a warning for passers-through. The crimson warts grew to the size of a large grape and hung from the victim's face and hands, lending the legend credence.

Travelers always planned to reach an inn by nightfall, but the dusk comes suddenly in the cold, foggy canyons and shelter wasn't always at hand. Then the flies would buzz softly, the fingers would envelop flesh, and the demon would examine its catch. If the victim was a stranger, the demon drew a shining ax and separated body from soul.

The Rímac River canyon was not a good route to the high deserts. But it was the only one.

On the switchbacks above the canyon, the llama trains wound back and forth, up the flank of the first chain of mountains. At the crest, the blue Pacific fell behind and the gray expanse of the high tableland, or *puna*, lay ahead. The switchbacks led down; the trail straightened and ran east through a lunar landscape of rocks and tufts of grass that waved in the cold wind.

The Indians and the llamas walked slowly, their chests expanding visibly with each deep breath. The altitude was fourteen thousand feet. It was a long way across the desert to La Oroya, hard against the second chain of peaks.

Most of the llama trains stopped there, but a few passed through La Oroya and took the trail north, toward Cerro de Pasco. That was where Daniel Carrión was born.

The first thing that marked him as special was his Spanish genes. He had Indian ones, too, but in his high world it was the Spanish blood that counted. His father, Baltazar Carrión, was both a lawyer and a medical doctor. His mother, Dolores Guerrero, was a celebrated beauty. But the attribute that most firmly set the boy apart was intelligence, coupled with a curious nature.

Also, there was the important matter of Castilian pride.

When he was a child, the legend goes, an important citizen of Cerro de Pasco remarked that Daniel's extraordinary grades owed more to his social status than to his keen mind. In time this statement was repeated to Daniel himself. He was outraged.

When the term ended and the students were called one by one before a jury of teachers to answer questions, Carrión passed easily and then convinced the jury to give him a copy of the questions. He took the sheet to his accuser and demanded that the man reexamine him personally, on the spot. The man asked the questions. The boy answered them promptly, precisely, correctly.

This proud and precocious boy was a child of his time, and his nature matched the Peruvian national character. Peru itself had glimpsed greatness. The world's richest nitrate deposits had been discovered to the south and, since nitrate was the basis for gunpowder, the find brought fantasies of world power. If Lima could control the gunpowder market, it could direct the armies of distant Europe.

There was even talk of a railroad into the *puna*, talk that crystallized when Daniel was twelve. The government hired a Yankee engineer, Henry Meiggs, to build a railroad from Lima to La Oroya. The line would run up the Rímac River valley, cross the Rímac once, tunnel beneath the peak, and stretch across the *puna* to La Oroya.

The hopes of the aristocracy, which included the Carrión family, rode high on this venture. The Railway to the Moon, as it was called, was to be Peru's great unifying force, bringing the same wealth to Peru that the transcontinental railway was bringing to the United States. The rails would carry untold riches from the high *puna* and the engine's whistle would arouse the Indian from his ancient lethargy.

Chileans who had helped build a similar railroad into the high country of their own nation were hired to carve the roadbed and lay the track from the coast to the tree line. Beyond that, the work would be done by Indian labor. By late 1871 there was service from Lima all the way to San Bartolomé at the mouth of the Rímac canyon. The work gangs pressed higher.

And the Chileans began to die.

It began with a fever. Then came the pain, waves of agony that bent the body double and left it screaming mindlessly. The temperature rose steadily as the pulse became rapid, weak, and irregular. The disease built slowly and subjective aeons elapsed before coma soothed the pain. Death slipped in quietly.

Railroad officials, refusing to believe the reports, rode to the end of the valley to watch the coffins come down. Then, comprehending the magnitude of the impending economic disaster, they ordered doctors to the railhead. The doctors quickly produced an elaborate description of the disease.

The valley was an awful place, they told the railroad executives. Sometimes, when a patient survived the fever and finally began to recover, he was afflicted with the damnable red warts that plagued the superstitious people who inhabited the place.

Having described the disease, the doctors named it Oroya fever, in dubious honor of the railway's destination. The name was to become synonymous with national mismanagement, wanton disregard for human life, and the inflexible stubbornness of power.

Up along the Rímac, the railroad crews continued to sicken and die. The doctors who named the disease said they could do nothing—Oroya fever wasn't even in the textbooks. So the railroad officials sent more construction workers. More bodies came down. More labor went up.

There was a desperate mutiny and the aristocrats dispatched the Army to put it down.

After the mutiny, the surviving Chilean workers slipped out of the camps at night, making their way downhill and south, fleeing the valley. Chinese slaves were purchased and led up the Rímac to replace them.

The track was to cross the river once, high in the valley. The engineers ordered a prefabricated bridge from the United States and the Chinese, many of them already sick, were instructed to assemble it across a chasm 575 feet wide. Two hundred and fifty-three feet below, the white river writhed against the boulders.

Daily the coffins came down. Replacements passed them on the narrow road.

As the dead came down the bills went up. Slaves, even the diminutive Chinese, were expensive. Panic in the labor camps translated into inefficiency, and fever led to carelessness. Tools slid over precipices and had to be replaced. Poorly laid track had to be ripped up and laid again. Deadlines came and went, unmet. Soon Meiggs began issuing paper bonds on the strength of the Peruvian government's backing.

The Chinese slaves erected the bridge, and one man died for each crosstie. The survivors named it the Bridge of Death. A smaller bridge across a tributary of the Rímac became known as the Bridge of Little Hell.

The line of track was laid, in the end, precisely as specified in the blueprints, and as an engineering feat it stood, and stands today, as a marvel of the hemisphere. But by the time the Railway to the Moon reached the high passes, Peru had squandered her treasury and, it is said, seven thousand human lives.

When the great national dream of the railroad was finally completed decades later, it belonged to British investors. Peru was already suffering at the hands of the mountain fever when Daniel Carrión reached the impressionable age of fourteen.

Though Daniel was socially removed from the sons of the Indian miners, he breathed the same rarefied air, shivered through the same frigid nights, and grew, small like the Indian miners, in the embrace of the *soroche*.

The *soroche*, or altitude sickness, enveloped the limbs and tore at the heart. The lungs heaved for air. Nausea convulsed the intestines and lethargy penetrated the marrow of the bones. The slow, calm movements of the Indians reflect the ancestral wisdom of a race that survived the *soroche* for three hundred centuries before the appearance of the Spaniards.

There is a *soroche* of the psyche as well. The high life is precarious, full of cold cliff faces and rope bridges that sway above boiling rivers. There, a stillness enfolds the mind and the shapes of companions and llamas fade into flat silhouettes of stone. The highlands teach the craftsmanship of brute survival, and the lessons can crush the mind, sap the will, and extinguish the pride.

The *puna* wasn't considered a fitting environment for the maturing offspring of conquistadores, so Daniel Carrión, at age fifteen, was packed off to Lima for an education and some city polish.

For older generations of tableland aristocrats, the journey to high school in Lima had been a test of manhood and an introduction to courage, but Daniel Carrión was the first of a new era. Just a few months before, the railroad that destroyed a treasury had reached Ticlio, near the summit. Daniel trekked across the *puna*, climbed the backside of the pass, and descended to the railhead.

There, where the big steam engines screamed and hissed and their whistles echoed sharply from the bare glacial amphitheaters, the frontier boy met modern technology. He jumped at the sudden blasts of live steam as the black monster machine came to a stop. Ticket gripped in his small hand, he climbed aboard and scrambled for a window seat.

Winding downward, the train looped back and forth, back and forth, back and forth. The air lost its purple hue, becoming whiter than Daniel had ever seen it. His ears ached and popped as the rock slid by, inches from his window. As the train crossed the famous Bridge of Death he looked down and his stomach rolled.

Several times the train stopped and a wretched Rímac Valley dweller got on the train. Some of them had huge, pendulous red warts hanging from their hands, their faces . . . even their ears.

The journey made an indelible impression on the adolescent's mind. Not long after, he vowed to a classmate that he would "make an important contribution to aching humanity."

At the National College of Guadalupe, where Carrión enrolled in high school, Daniel continued to earn the best grades in his class. There he grew to his full height of just over four feet. His nose became sharp as his olive face lost its adolescent fat and became set in a serious expression.

He didn't make friends easily, but those he made he kept, and when he enrolled in San Marcos University for premedical training in the natural sciences he took a band of the high school's best students with him.

History records their names as Casimiro Medina, Enrique Mestanza, Julian Arce, Mariano Alcedan, Ricardo Miranda, and Manuel Montero. When in 1879 Daniel Carrión entered the university's medical school, the second oldest in the New World, he was again accompanied in the enrollment lines by his friends.

As they and Carrión studied in high school and college, their generation's most precious national dreams collapsed around them. Work ceased on the Railroad to Poverty.

The nitrate mines proved more difficult to develop than
had been anticipated. And the rival nation to the south,
Chile, threatened to steal the dreams so carefully nurtured
in Lima.

For years, Chilean companies had worked nitrate mines
along Bolivia's desert coastland, the territory that connected inland Bolivia to the sea and separated the boundaries of Chile and Peru.

Chile was an efficient democracy and, under her control, the Bolivian mines were fiercely competitive, out-
producing and underselling Peru's. Chile's railroad was a
spectacular success. Decisions made in Santiago began to
reverberate through the throne rooms of Europe.

Alarmed by Chile's growing power, Bolivia and Peru
secretly signed a mutual defense pact. Soon Bolivia, urged
on by Peru, levied a heavy export tax on the Chilean nitrate companies. In Santiago, businessmen talked war.

In the year Daniel Carrión entered medical school, the
Chilean Army occupied Bolivia's entire seacoast province
while the Chilean Navy sailed north to blockade the Peruvian ports of Iquique and Arica. Soon most of Peru's war-
ships had been sunk or, worse, captured.

As Carrión was settling down to his medical books, the
last Peruvian ship dipped its colors to the overpowering
Chilean forces and Peru of the golden dreams lay open to
the enemy fleet. The Chilean Army began to move.

News of fighting far to the south reached Lima and circulated through the university dormitories, where the elite
of Peruvian manhood passed rumors and pledged alle-
giance to their country. The Bolivian troops fell back before superior cannon and seasoned troops.

In 1881 the masts of the enemy Navy appeared offshore
and thousands of students, Daniel Carrión among them,
ran to the southern shores of the city to drive back the
landing parties. But the defenders were amateurs, armed

only with primitive weapons, soft hands, and good intentions. When the Battle of Miraflores was finished a significant portion of Peru's intellectual future lay dead on the field. The president of the country fled to Colombia in shame.

Daniel and his friends survived, but their identities were forever altered. The footfall of the invader echoed in the National Library. Chilean infantrymen slept in the ornate halls of San Marcos University. Cut off from the outside world, family wealth evaporated. Food was scarce, poverty ubiquitous, suffering acute. First-generation immigrants to Lima, mostly Indians who had come to better their social status, fled at the first opportunity. The surrender, when it came, stripped Bolivia of her only access to the sea and forfeited all of the south of Peru, including the nitrate fields.

Daniel Carrión's country was broken but Daniel Carrión was not. He turned to his studies.

As he became absorbed in the diseases of his people, he read about the red warts that he had seen in the Rímac Valley. There was much written, but little said.

Peruvian warts, as they were known, constituted an awful disease that was sometimes fatal. A fever struck first; then the ugly excrescences appeared, hanging even from the nostrils and ears. In 1845 its cause was pronounced by a certain Dr. Tschudi to be wells and springs contaminated with a substance called wart-water. He said a drop of wart-water produced one wart; two drops produced two warts; and so on. He identified the contaminated wells and for thirty years the people of the valley avoided them, but the warts came anyway.

Then a Dr. Dounon challenged the theory decisively by touring the valley with two assistants, methodically drinking from all the wells Dr. Tschudi said were contaminated. History doesn't record whether or not Dr.

Dounon had a theory of his own, but the trio didn't develop a single wart among them.

In 1874 a Dr. Raimondi claimed that poisonous frogs caused the warts. The next year Dr. Pancorvo said fumes from the soil caused them. Two years later Dr. Tupper argued that the disease was due to a "miasmatic agent."

Carrión, true to his studies of scientific principles, was puzzled that none of the doctors offered any scientific evidence for their theories. The only convincing data, in fact, came from Dr. Dounon, who had drunk the well-water. And he hadn't advanced any theory at all.

As for the present, Carrión soon became fascinated with a dispute on the nature of warts between two of the hemisphere's premier physician-scientists. Dr. Salazar, a Peruvian, advanced a theory that Peruvian warts were, in fact, the same disease as Oroya fever. The opposing view came from a Chilean, Dr. Izquierdo, who wrote that the diseases were separate and very distinct. Warts were one thing, he asserted, and the fever that had crippled the Railway to the Moon was something else, probably nothing more than malaria. It just happened that some victims were luckless enough, or wretched enough, to get both diseases. Eventually, as all noted physician-scientists along the Pacific coast did, Dr. Izquierdo visited San Marcos University. A lecture was scheduled. Carrión and his friends were there.

According to the legend of Daniel Carrión, the medical student listened to the noted doctor in silence—but when the presentation was finished the young man was on his feet demanding evidence. It was a surprising ploy. Professors of that era were not accustomed to the questions of students.

The physician recovered his poise quickly, however, and answered that evidence was superfluous. After all, he, Dr. Izquierdo, a scientist of wide fame and unquestionable authority, had clearly stated that warts and fever were separate diseases. Did the student think he, who was not yet even a doctor, could state the fact more eloquently? Had the student's pride gotten the better of his respect? The class laughed.

Carrión sat down, his face hot with embarrassment.

Later, alone in his room, Carrión decided that Dr. Izquierdo, having no evidence, was a fraud. Apparently his rival, Dr. Salazar, was correct. Warts and fever must be a single disease. The perception that the Peruvian scientist was superior to the Chilean one gave Carrión satisfaction.

When a lecture was scheduled by Dr. Salazar, Carrión was in the front row. Again he listened respectfully but Dr. Salazar, like Dr. Izquierdo, offered no evidence. Carrión mortified his friends by repeating the earlier spectacle. His question was the same. The answer wasn't different enough to matter, and the laughter was familiar, too. Some of it came from his friends.

Disgusted and believing himself disgraced, Carrión washed his hands of the theories and went back to the study of warts. Soon he would be allowed to see real patients. He would ask his own questions. They were Peruvian questions, he told his friends, and they must be answered by a Peruvian scientist.

By 1882, when Carrión treated his first patient, he had already begun to plan the work that he hoped would later earn him a doctorate. He chose to study warts, of course. Specifically, he would investigate the early symptoms of the disease, about which little was known.

The medical ignorance about the early manifestations of Peruvian warts stemmed, as is so often the case, from lack of proximity. The doctors were down in the city. The patients were out in the boondocks.

Peruvian wart patients were brought to the hospital only after their disease had progressed to the point of imminent danger to life. Then the thin, bony bodies were put on litters and aboard the train. They entered the hospital with high fevers, heads bobbing insanely, eyes protruding, lips forming dissociated words. Warts hung from every part of their bodies. The disease usually wasn't fatal, but most of the patients whom doctors saw in the hospital were already fated to die. It was too late for herb poultices, purgatives, and bleeding.

Carrión knew vaguely that the warts were preceded by a fever, but little else was known of the early stages. Perhaps if the illness could be recognized earlier, the physicians in the valley might be able to treat it sooner with better results.

How could the early symptoms of Peruvian warts be defined? That would be Carrión's question, and the means to an answer seemed self-apparent. Like Dr. Dounon, who dared to drink the wart-water, Carrión would be his own experimental subject. He would experience the disease himself, taking careful notes.

Carrión discussed this idea with his friends. They were less than impressed and didn't hide the fact. They said self-experimentation was stupid.

"What about it?" Carrión argued, in the passionate syntax of his native language. "I'm not frightened by the skin deformities, and if the disease develops so seriously that it affects a vital organ, I'm ready to pay with my life.

"Besides," he added, "it bothers me to see a doctor like the Chilean Izquierdo, who has only seen a few tumors and goes around giving opinions and writing about a disease which nobody is better qualified than us to discuss. With the exception of the work of Doctors Salazar and Velez, I have not heard of any other studies by compatriots of this problem.

"You know that I've had enough time to think about this . . . that I've considered ahead of time the serious consequences that it could have for me. But is not medicine advanced in great part due to risky experimentation?

"Then why be distrustful?" he asked. "The results, in any case, must be good."

Still, he hesitated. The arguments of his friends, the pressures of school and clinic, the occasional trips home . . . time passed. But at the end of the day Daniel Carrión would lie in his rooming house bed exhausted, and his fatigued mind would drift back to the warts and the superior air of the Chilean.

Then, in 1885, the Free Academy of Medicine established a prize for important discoveries concerning Peruvian warts. In Europe, several well-known scientists became intrigued by the problem and sent to San Marcos University for tissue samples. Daniel Carrión went into a frenzy. A Peruvian, not a foreigner, not a foreigner, *not a foreigner* must win the prize.

The date was August 27. Because of the season, only one active case of Peruvian warts was in the hospital and that patient, though he still had a wart over his right eye, was ready for discharge. Carrión slipped a thin, sharp lancet into his pocket and rushed to the ward. As it became clear what was about to happen, other doctors and at least two professors gathered.

They all counseled against the experiment, but no one raised a hand to stop it.

In the excitement, Carrión was awkward. His shaking hands were unable to handle the lancet, and he fumbled badly. A young doctor in the group now stepped forward and took the sharp instrument. Expertly he jabbed it first into the wart and then into Carrión's arm. Once. Twice. Three times. Four. Drops of blood appeared on the puncture wounds. Carrión stared at his arm. The spectators began to disperse. In the flesh of Carrión's arm, in the layer of fat beneath the skin, tiny bacteria wriggled in the bloodstream.

They were mere specks of microbes, twenty-five thou-

sand of them to an inch, a size that suited them to existence in the entrails of the small sand fly that, according to
legend, accompanied the invisible demon in the valley of
the Rímac. The human body was foreign territory, but
the bacteria survived. One attached itself to a passing red
blood cell and burrowed inside.

The medical student opened his notebook. "The inocu-
lations were done with the blood that had been taken from
a wart located on the right frontal sinus region of the patient Carmen Paredes in bed number five of Our Lady of
Mercy Hospital. . . ."

Then he waited.

Busy days passed. There were studies, questions to answer, patients to tend in the clinic, more studies, more
questions. A week passed. Two. In his veins, in the para-
sitized red blood cell, many bacteria now grew, rod-
shaped ones, C-shaped ones, and others that looked like
the letter X. Slowly, the membrane of the blood cell rup-
tured, spilling a new generation of bacteria into the flow-
ing blood. On September 17, exactly three weeks after the
inoculation, Daniel wrote in his notebook that he felt
tired. The next day he experienced pains in his left ankle.
But those things were vague and the discomfort passed.
He continued his schedule.

On September 19, he sat at his desk, absorbed in his
studies. The flame in the lamp flickered periodically. A
Pacific breeze came through a window of the old rooming
house, and a curtain moved. Carrión turned a page.

The pain came without warning.

Carrión bent double, his head striking the desk, the
book skittering across the floor. He clenched his teeth and
waited, not moving, his mind clear, collecting data. Motion made it worse; he knew that from experience in the
clinic. His face glistened with sweat. Eventually his heavy
breathing grew more regular and his fingers moved along

the desk toward the notebook. The hands of the clock turned to midnight and beyond.

"September 20. The pains become almost unbearable. I am able to remain in the same position for not more than a brief moment; continually, I twist and change my place on the bed without obtaining the slightest comfort or rest. During the night my temperature has risen to 103.6 degrees."

Summoned by the landlady, Carrión's friends gathered around his bed. They tried to feed him, but he couldn't eat. Sweat slid down the planes of his body and onto the bed and Carrión shivered in the soaked sheets. He craved water. His urine turned dark red. His hands gripped the notebook.

"September 21. . . . My temperature is now 104.9 degrees. Everything else remains unchanged.

"September 22. . . . Red spots like fleabites have appeared, some on the nose, others on the right cheekbone and between the eyebrows. Otherwise, there are the same pains and discomforts which continue as before.

"September 23. . . . Especially severe pains in the right shoulder, arm and elbow. . . .

"September 24. . . . The right hand soon becomes fatigued and stiff. . . . The left hand, though unaccustomed . . . must be used for writing.

"September 25. . . . Stiffness has spread to the forefingers of both hands. . . . Writing becomes even more difficult than before. . . ."

Hour by hour, the multiplying bacteria destroyed the blood cells. Oxygen ceased to flow freely to the organs of the body and Carrión writhed in agony, vomited, discharged fetid liquid from his bowels. The thirst was terrible.

The young scientist feverishly counseled his friends to relax. Soon the warts would appear, the fever would break, and there would be a long period of recovery. The students seemed to agree. They tended him constantly.

Deep lines appeared in his face and his eyes began to protrude, showing white all around the pupils. The students discovered a murmur developing in the bottom of his heart.

September 26. . . . "Beginning today my friends will write down my observations for me, which I must confess I find most difficult. . . ." The penmanship of the remaining notes changed periodically as Carrión's friends sat by the bed, each in turn, copying down the pertinent observations. They endured a steady barrage of abuse from the patient, who repeatedly accused them of recording too little detail.

"He complains mostly of his pains," one note-taker wrote, "and of a continuous sensation of vertigo that prevents him from making the slightest movement. He often grows angry because he cannot sleep nor can he sit up without experiencing the most extreme nausea. He has no appetite; upon our continued insistence, he has eaten a bit of food and swallowed a small amount of wine. He makes frequent convulsive movements. . . .

"September 28. . . . Severe anemic condition . . . most serious . . . The cardiac tremors increase alarmingly. No sign of warts."

His friends prayed.

"October 1. . . . He has averted death only through his own indomitable will, yet he refuses our aid in his bodily needs. He tells us, laughing, 'You take alarm too readily and stare fearfully at me as if I were already on my way to the graveyard.'"

As Daniel Carrión's body weakened, his mind shuffled and recataloged the symptoms—and still, after all this time, no warts. The symptoms were worse than he had anticipated, and grimly familiar. From the blood of a wart, he had contracted Oroya fever.

Peruvian warts and Oroya fever were the same disease. Izquierdo, the Chilean, was a fool. Carrión, the Peruvian, had demonstrated Izquierdo's error for the world to see.

On October 3 a medical school doctor arrived in the room, insisting that Carrión go to the hospital for a blood transfusion. Carrión refused.

". . . His skin is turned dry like old parchment and is of a light-yellow hue. Gums and lips are completely pale and have the appearance of wax discolored by candle smoke. The facial aspect is disfigured; cheeks and temples are deeply hollowed; the nose is sharp and the ears translucent. The eyes sink deep into the sockets and each is surrounded by a dark circle; they are shadowy and dull, little remaining of their former brightness and vivacity. Nothing is left, even in moments of extreme animation, of the vigor and enthusiasm he once possessed in abundance."

Daniel Carrión, as dying Oroya fever victims often did, heard the frantic pulse beat through the large arteries of his neck. Repeatedly he touched his fingers to his throat, feeling, as he had been trained, for that grim, rattling throb. He changed his mind about the hospital, and his friends carried the stretcher.

That evening his mind slid beneath the rising fever and his lips babbled of warts, and fevers, and parents, and snowcapped mountains, and Peru.

According to the records, Carrión's mind cleared suddenly at 11:30 P.M. on October 5, 1885. He turned to Enrique Mestanza.

"Enrique," Carrión said in French. "It's over."

Shortly his breathing ceased. Enrique stood slowly, as did the rest.

There were no warts on the shriveled body they wrapped and laid in the wooden coffin. Warts, Carrión knew before he died, were a sign of blessing, of recovery, and they appeared only on the flesh of the fortunate.

Oroya fever was the deadly precursor of warts.

The people in the valley, with an immunity caused by long exposure, weathered the fever and developed the warts. Outsiders didn't live long enough.

Daniel Carrión's friends carried the coffin slowly through the streets of Lima. Up through the Maison de Sante the coffin moved slowly, followed by two hundred mourners, through the Plazuela de San Carlos, through the Plazuela de la Inquisición, along the road in front of the university, into the cemetery. One disease, not two.

The Chilean was in error.

Carrión's dramatic experiment focused national attention on the scourge of the valley of the Rímac and challenged the country's medical men to find the answer. Within twenty years of his death another Peruvian, Alberto Barton, focused his microscope on the elusive bacteria that had destroyed the dream of a Railway to the Moon.

Early in the new century scientists reached the same conclusion as the people of the Rímac Valley; in 1912 the dusk-flying sand fly, with or without accompanying demon, was shown to be the carrier of the disease. Mosquito netting became the prevention and, after the Second World War, penicillin became the cure.

But more than a single scientific discovery is required to explain the honor that has accrued to the young scientist in the century since his death. He gave science a fact, but he gave his country something more.

It was a Peruvian problem, he had asserted, and a Peruvian must solve it. A defeated, bankrupt people found pride in that and a young man who might have been called a fool in another time became, instead, a martyr.

Today Carrión is the patron saint of Peruvian science. An idealized likeness of his stern face gazes across the Daniel Carrión School of Medicine in Lima. The notes he and his friends kept so faithfully are preserved as a national treasure by the trustees of San Marcos University.

There, in the shadow of the Andes, historians as well as medical students study the curse of the Rímac Valley and the courageous discovery of the affliction known as Carrión's disease.

THE LAST OF THE MIASMATISTS

The year 1818 was an auspicious one in ways that would not become clear for generations. In Bavaria, where the Pettenkofer family lived with its newborn son, a constitution was signed. In neighboring Germany, another new father and mother chose the name Karl, Karl for commoner, Karl for man of the people—Karl Marx. In Stockholm, Baron Jöns Jakob Berzelius published a book listing the molecular weights of two thousand compounds and labored over his theory that chemicals combined in accordance with a property he called "valences." In England, nine-year-old Charles Darwin trudged through the grammar of Latin, not yet fascinated by the myriad shapes of beetles.

But it wasn't the slow dawn of a new age that governed the lives of the Pettenkofer family and its newest member. Their ancestry was one of serfdom fading into poverty, and the new infant's healthy cries were also hungry ones. He was another mouth to feed and the immediate future was frightening and uncertain.

At the time Bavaria was ruled by King Maximilian I, and so Max was a hopeful name for the baby—a wistful name, perhaps, but one that might somehow bless and aid the child who carried it. And so the shopkeeper and his

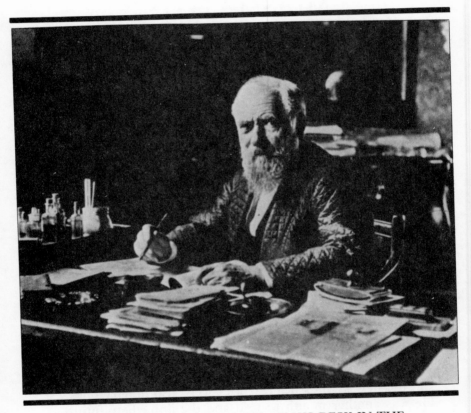

DR. MAX VON PETTENKOFER AT HIS DESK IN THE
HYGIENIC INSTITUTE

Courtesy Dr. Hermann Eyer of the Max von Pettenkofer Institute, Munich

wife, knowing they could offer their latest child little else, gave him a royal name.

In that year, adding to the more familiar fears of disease and violence, there were rumors of a mysterious plague that moved across the distant East. According to travelers, it began like the common cholera nostra, an unpleasant but far from deadly diarrhea that could keep a man out of the fields for a day or two. But the diarrhea that raged in the East was explosive and struck like a hammer. Strong men rose in the morning, in apparent health, and by nightfall they lay dead in their own watery excretions.

It had started in India, in the pesthole of Calcutta, and now it crept unseen, unstoppable, across the countryside. Because it involved diarrhea it was called cholera, but not cholera nostra.

Cholera morbus, the doctors said, "the cholera of death."

Or just "the cholera."

The Pettenkofer parents waited for the death to come, and like their countrymen, rich and poor, they prayed to God to spare them and their children.

Their prayers were answered. The great tide of cholera lapped at the doorstep of Moscow in 1822, and then its advance faltered. It receded to the East, toward its homeland, India.

In the meantime life, though precious, was difficult. The infant Max Pettenkofer learned to walk and was assigned chores. In the winter, the Alpine snows lay across the valley of the Danube and cold was synonymous with hunger, or the fear of hunger. The peasant farmers had little money to spend at the Pettenkofer store. Max's father labored over his books, trying to figure out how to make ends meet. The trouble was that he had too many children.

The shopkeeper had a more successful brother, Franz,

who lived in Munich. Franz was a chemist and had secured an appointment as apothecary to the king. The shopkeeper hesitated, then reached for pen and paper.

In Munich, Franz read the letter sympathetically. He paid special attention to his brother's description of young Max. The lad was precocious, a good reader, good at sums, willing, capable . . .

Franz visited his brother's family and was introduced to the ten-year-old. The boy looked up at him soberly, and answered his uncle's questions quickly and accurately. Clearly, Franz decided, his brother was right. Young Max was a bright child and should take easily to the demands of apprenticeship. Max sat stiffly beside his uncle as the carriage horse clip-clopped toward the distant city and a new life.

Franz treated Max like one of his own many children and even, at times, doted on him. The child was quick to master the mortar and pestle, proved eager to learn, and exhibited a stubborn perfectionism that made him especially suited to the apothecary's trade. Later, with training, the lad would be a chemist. Not a mere apothecary, but a real chemist.

For his part, Max recognized the opportunity he had been offered, and he seized it.

The mortar was a deep dish made of stone and the heavy, clublike pestle fitted into it. The grinding motion was back and forth, back and forth, around and around, around and around. Slowly, the seeds and crystals turned to a flour that adhered to the sides of the mortar.

The apothecary shop was neat and clean. The walls were lined with drawers that came up to Max's chest, and above those were shelves that reached the ceiling and contained hundreds and hundreds of matched jars. There was a ladder for the apprentices to climb on as they scampered about the shop, refilling this, fetching that, mixing, grinding.

It was an orderly world, in which everything was carefully labeled. There was cinchona bark from Peru, which contained quinine, useful for malaria. There was cumin from Egypt, spikenard from Java, cinnamon from Ceylon, currants from Greece, galingale from Malay, datura from Bengal.

All these things came in boxes, kegs, and sacks with foreign writing on them, and most of them ultimately had to be ground into powders by the junior apprentice. Max stood for hours, rhythmically moving the pestle.

He learned the recipes by heart. Black draught consisted of senna, currants, coriander seed, cream of tartar, and manna from the flowering ash. It loosened the bowels. So did compound licorice powder, which was a mixture of senna, licorice, caraway, fennel, cumin, spikenard, cinnamon, galingale, and gromwell seeds.

In fact, many of the preparations were for laxatives. Purging was the one thing that doctors could offer and so, when in doubt, they offered it.

As for the rumored cholera . . . once again, the travelers said, it advanced through Russia. There were stories that the czar, attempting to stifle the advance, had sent troops to surround the infected villages and shoot anyone who attempted to leave. But the cholera gripped the soldiers and jumped through their lines to still another town. By 1830, as young Max was just beginning to learn the skills of an apprentice apothecary, it was in Moscow.

The doctors of Munich discussed the new advance, but they were as impotent as they had been when the Black Death devastated the city five hundred years earlier. And like the Black Death, cholera was apparently caused by a miasma—something spread by air, a deadly poison that couldn't be stopped. Along with the rest of the populace, the doctors attended church and begged God to spare their city once again.

No one talked about cholera in front of the children, of

course, but the children eavesdropped, as children do. Max knew, in an abstract way, about the death that seized Moscow.

But where was Moscow? To an apothecary's apprentice, faraway Moscow was printing on a bottle of caviar. Life was here, in Munich, at the center of the world, dressed in lace like a lady of the court, echoing in the ringing words of the writer Johann Wolfgang von Goethe.

King Max had died shortly before his country namesake became an apprentice apothecary in Munich, and had been replaced on the throne by Ludwig I, a fine and sensitive king who patronized the arts and encouraged them in Munich. Thanks to his good graces, the common people heard the dramatic words of the best playwrights of the era.

While visiting the court and performing on outdoor wooden stages, artists, actors, composers, and philosophers often found themselves ill and in need, perhaps, of a laxative. Or their elegant, lacy ladies requested sulfur, mixed with ointment, to paint on their rashes.

The apprentice stood patiently at the mortar, grinding the yellow sulfur crystals beneath the pestle, daydreaming. Munich was the center of the cultural world and it was only natural, only right, that God had again answered the people's prayers. Cholera reigned in England now, and across the Atlantic, in New York, a hundred people died each day, but in Munich violins played the music of Ludwig van Beethoven and actors amused the court with the words of Faust. Along with his cousins Max went to hear plays and concerts, and the ringing voices and haunting music affected him deeply.

The adolescent was captivated by the culture that flowed around him, but he tried to keep his attention where it belonged, which was on his studies. He learned how chemicals combined in the order of their valences, and he was fascinated by the orderliness of science. He was honestly interested in the phenomena he encountered, the way two things could combine to create a third thing, different in all ways from the first two. Sodium sulfide, for instance, was a powdery, odorless substance. But when hydrochloric acid was poured over it, it was somehow activated and it turned into a putrid-smelling gas that duplicated the stench of rotten eggs.

Out of love, gratitude, and duty he dreamed his uncle's dream of becoming a chemist, and he was honestly interested in his own right, too. But as he stood measuring potions for an artistic and enlightened court, a heretical fantasy intruded into his mind. How wonderful it would be to be an actor. An apothecary's life was dull and routine, but an actor . . . an actor could travel, escort beautiful ladies to masked balls, converse with kings, make a mark in the world!

Of course, Max knew he never could be an actor. It was his destiny to seize the opportunity that was granted him, to bloom where he was planted. He would be a chemist. But he wished . . .

In the daytime he went to school. At night he worked between the lonely dry shelves while the fantasy nagged and pulled at him. The fantasy grew into a wish, and that into a need. He concealed the guilty thing from his uncle, but couldn't resist finally stammering it out to his sympathetic cousin, the tiny, pretty Helene.

Sometimes, when he was alone—or almost alone—he recited Goethe. He tried his hand at sonnets. Helene admired the results.

It was an idyllic dream in an idyllic city in an idyllic time, but the forces at work in the world were brutal. In 1835, Halley's comet appeared in the sky. The following year, the summer that Max was eighteen, cholera again swept across Russia—and this time it invaded Munich with a vengeance.

As in other cities, the epidemic began in the slums and throughout the siege of death the poor suffered most. Cartwrights and their wives, laborers and laundresses, beggars and prostitutes died first by the dozens, then the hundreds. Terror gripped the city and there was panic in the streets.

It was worse, even, than the travelers had reported. The first symptom might be no more than a surprised look as the victim's bowels emptied without warning, soiling his garments. If the cholera struck in the street, people drew back in horror.

It had been rumored to kill quickly, but for the victim it wasn't quick enough. The surprise changed to agony as he was hit by a cramping pain that set him writhing on the bed. Copious quantities of watery liquid poured through his anus, fouling the mattress.

As the pain intensified over the hours, the patient drew up into a ball, chin against knees, breath whistling softly between his teeth. When the victim died at this stage, which he often did, the body couldn't be unrolled and had to be buried in the fetal position.

Those who survived the first attack then faced, after a night of agony, a slow recovery or, more often, an equally slow decline into death. The patient's cheeks became hollow as his bodily liquids surged, more weakly now but still beyond control, onto the bedclothes, carrying tiny fragments of his colon with it. As the hours became days his skin darkened and his eyes stared vacantly, without comprehension and, finally, without life.

Throughout the city, harried physicians rushed from sickbed to sickbed with their lancets and leeches. Carpenters and cabinetmakers were fully employed, and the price of coffins soon became so outrageous that the poor had to wrap the blackened bodies of their beloved dead in blankets and sheets. Screaming and crying, tattered remnants of families followed the body carts through the otherwise deserted streets.

The cholera raged mostly among the poor, but it killed the rich often enough that the terror gripped the entire city, sparing no one. The cholera traveled in the air, it was said—a miasma. The windows of the palace were kept tightly shut. The schools closed and Max labored in the pharmacy, concocting bouquets of lavender, mint, balm, chamomile, sweet flag, rue, and peppermint, to be held beneath the frightened noses of the royalty.

If death disrupted the routine of the poor, economic and social disaster threatened the rich. Bizarre rumors circulated. A woman, passed by a funeral cortege, had felt the dread cholera pass from the body of the dead man into her own and a few hours later she was dead. Death stalked you, chose you, and closed around you. It was everywhere. Thousands set out walking, fleeing the city, disrupting commerce.

The city fathers pleaded with those fleeing the blighted city. . . . Running wouldn't help, they said. Cholera wasn't contagious. If it were contagious, the czar would have been able to stop it with soldiers. Cholera was a miasma breathed equally by all, and if you had breathed it, it wouldn't help to run. It was already in you.

The authorities pleaded with the populace to stay where they were, but they minimized the disease's class distinctions, and whenever possible they denied that the distinction even existed. When the plague had struck Hungary, the poor, having heard of Malthus's teachings, had concluded that cholera was caused by a conspiracy to reduce their numbers; therefore they had staged a bloody uprising. So the disease's preference for the poor was talked about only behind the closed doors of the aristocracy, where the doctors reasoned that the causes were filth, laziness, and neglected hygiene.

Finally, as the weeks passed, the air grew cold, and the snow line marched down the Bavarian Alps, the deaths tapered off and the cholera was gone. There were more cases the following spring, but the epidemic was far less severe. The number of cases would continue to dwindle, but Pettenkofer's Munich would never again be totally free of the disease.

The glittering life of the court never returned to its previous glory, either. There was a nasty story that good King Ludwig was under the spell of the beautiful schemer Lola Montez, and that he ran the government at her bidding. As the king grew middle-aged amid the murmur of scandal, he began to lose his liberal bent and his policies grew increasingly reactionary. In the apothecary shop, Max Pettenkofer quarreled with his uncle. He would be an actor, the young man vowed, jutting out his chin defiantly.

Helene tried desperately to mediate, but Max was stubborn and her father, Franz, was implacable. Angrily Max stormed out of his adopted home to join a band of traveling actors.

Life was difficult for a beginning actor but Max's incessant secret practicing in the apothecary shop and behind the house paid off. He was cold and hungry sometimes, and life in a traveling company entailed as much muscle work as oratorical skill. But here for the first time the young man's genius took hold, and soon reviewers were praising his extraordinary histrionic ability.

In Goethe's *Egmont* he played the part of Brackenburg, tortured by a desperate and unrequited love for the manipulative Clara. Driven to the brink of suicide, he held a vial of poison before him. The worst sadness, he shouted to the gods and the audience, was the sadness of dashed hopes.

"Could I but forget the time that she loved me, seemed

to love me. . . . She seemed to soften, she looked at me, my brain reeled, I felt her lips on mine, and—now? Die, wretch! Why dost thou hesitate?"

But as Goethe's Brackenburg found that he lacked the courage to drink the poison, Max Pettenkofer discovered that he didn't possess that indefinable quality that drives an aspiring artist to persevere. Or perhaps the frustrating chaos of the arts, once it enfolded him, didn't have the potential he had thought. Perhaps he perceived, with distance from the mortar and pestle, that those tools were far more powerful than he had given them credit for being. History doesn't say.

Again Helene intervened as a peacemaker and, this time, he allowed himself to be cajoled into coming home. Uncle Franz wrote off the affair as an incident of youthful rebellion and welcomed the errant young man home. Shortly after, Max obediently enrolled at the University of Munich to begin his formal study of chemistry.

Though he turned his back on acting, Max's sense of destiny and drama still burned hot. He had traded the stage for the laboratory, that was all. Mature now, he perceived that the most exciting drama unfolding in the world was on the stage of science, and the descendant of serfs was as determined as ever to succeed. He worked diligently at his studies and asked Helene for her hand. She accepted, and Uncle Franz blessed them. They would be wed, once Max had achieved a position in life.

Somehow, he promised Helene and himself, he would make his mark. When he wasn't studying he worked in the laboratory, trying things, mixing things—failing, mostly, as students do . . . but the world of science was young, and persistent curiosity and determination were quickly rewarded.

Before receiving his bachelor's degree he had published two scientific papers. One described a method used to test for the presence of arsenic, a procedure that would still be used by medical detectives a century later. The second detailed a technique for separating arsenic from antimony.

Though Max's interest was in the science of chemistry, there was no school for that in Munich, and as a matter of expediency he enrolled instead in a school intended to train doctors and surgeons. But he had no intention of actually practicing the healing arts. He especially would not be, God forbid, an apothecary.

When he received his degree in medicine and surgery in 1843, he counted his meager savings and told his uncle that he wanted to go to Giessen, to study under the famous biochemist Justus von Liebig. Full of hope, he wrote to Liebig. The reply was crushing. There was no room. Instead, Max was accepted in Würzburg, in the laboratory of Josef Scherer.

Scherer, like Liebig, was working in that hazy, borderline area between chemistry and physiology. Pettenkofer was attracted to the growing perception of man's body as somehow . . . almost . . . a chemical machine. It was a perception of life that made some nervous, but Newton, were he still alive, would have loved it. Biochemistry offered the medical profession a precision it had never before known, and it was a fertile area, rich in possibilities, one in which an ambitious young man with intelligence could do great works and go far.

It was also the most interesting thing that Max could imagine, more mesmerizing even than literature . . . though the young scientist still wrote a poem or two, when he had time. It was amazing, the beautiful balance of life. Chemicals entered through the mouth and lungs. The body did something to them, used them somehow, and then excreted what was left through the kidneys, bowels, and skin. What it excreted was different from what it consumed, as different as the rotten-smelling hydrogen sulfide was from the hydrochloric acid and sodium sulfide that combined to make it.

The environment was also chemical, so the body naturally reacted to it. If you gave a man arsenic, for instance, the chemical did something to the man, and he died. What mysterious thing it did to gum up the chemical works nobody knew, but the deed was surely chemical in nature. There obviously were other poisons, too . . . unknown ones. There were poisons, of some sort, in the miasmas that caused diseases like cholera.

If poisons were chemicals, that didn't make chemicals bad. Foods were chemicals, too, useful chemicals, and the body was very sensitive to them. Excrement was also chemicals, products of the food that had been eaten. For instance, Max discovered in the laboratory, there was an acid in the urine that could be measured and quantified. The amount varied, depending on what the person ate. Ecstatic over his first discovery as a bona fide chemist, Max wrote his findings in a paper that was quickly published.

The more he worked, the more Max was awed by the complexity of the chemical interactions between man and his environment. The idea fit nicely into the enduring theory that disease was caused by something in the air, perhaps a gas, a miasma. Some environments were unhealthy. . . .

Such reasoning was given added weight because the answers they provided fit easily into the human psyche. Even cats cleaned themselves. The poor lived in filthy surroundings, but that wasn't of their own choosing. What man, left to his own devices, would willingly live in filth, or dampness? Spoiled meat wasn't pleasant to eat. A draft was noxious. Dirty water tasted bad. . . .

That thought sent a shudder through his mind. In Munich, the public water was so bad that only the poor drank it. The burghers drank beer. Perhaps there were poisons in the water, which would explain why the poor suffered more from disease.

Max worked late hours in the laboratory, collecting bodily fluids and diluting them, mixing them with other things, pouring them from test tube to test tube, heating them. He taught himself as never before to think logically, rationally, carefully. He tried things. Mostly, he didn't understand the result, but sometimes, often enough to drive him on, he did.

He found something else, something strange, in the urine. It was nitrogen and . . . and something. What? Whatever it was, the amount varied.

Some of what he discovered was even useful. Another paper, this one describing a test for bile salts, appeared in print.

Now, in 1844, with four published papers to Max's credit, Liebig found there was room after all in Giessen. In glee, Max abandoned the Scherer laboratory and joined Liebig. If anything, he worked even harder.

But it was too late. His money was running out, his uncle was in poor health, and Helene was growing less patient. The time had come when Max had to quit studying and get a job. Not, of course, as an apothecary. In the same year he moved to Giessen he moved again, this time back to Munich, where he had secured a position in the royal mint. A wedding date was set.

At night, he pursued his research career. Saliva, he found, contained a compound called sulfocyanic acid. There was oxyproteic acid in urine.

And there was, for that matter, a lot of platinum in the gold used to make the crown thaler, the coin of Bavaria. Now, if you could only get the platinum out, the coins would be easier to make . . . and you'd have the platinum, besides. . . .

Max could have spent the rest of his life cataloging the different molecules that make up urine, and no king would have noticed him for his efforts. But when he discovered how to extract platinum from gold . . . when a young man improves the coin of the realm, well.

Max Pettenkofer? King Ludwig asked. Son of Franz, the royal apothecary? Oh. Not son. Nephew. Well, whoever he is, he'll go far.

In fact, the royal mind was better attuned to art and economics than to science. Take glass, for instance. Bavaria was famous for its quality glassware and naturally Ludwig prided himself on an eye for fine glass . . . like the wonderful red glass someone found in Pompeii. A shard had found its way into the king's hand. He examined it, held it to the light. The redness had an almost unearthy quality, and it was very, very beautiful.

If such glass could be duplicated in Bavaria it would create a great demand and increase employment in the northeast section of the country, where glass was manufactured. That would be nice, especially with the furor over Lola. The gossip made Ludwig tired. What was unusual about a king's taking a mistress if he wanted one? They just didn't understand how valuable she was to him.

The king looked at the glass again. How had it been made so beautifully, perfectly, translucently red?

Ludwig summoned a number of the country's most prestigious chemists and commissioned them to go to Pompeii, to find out. Several months later they came back without an answer. The king was chagrined.

Max wasn't on the commission, of course, since he wasn't a famous chemist. But he was a chemist nonetheless and he heard about the problem, and considered it. He liked challenges, and to pit himself against problems that had baffled others.

Red glass. The red came from an impurity of some sort.

Being red, like rust, it was probably some molecule based on iron . . . an oxide?

In the daytime, Max worked in the mint's lab, testing and assaying. At night, he worked on the glass. He was delighted to find that yes, he had guessed correctly. The molecule, whatever it was, was based on iron.

A few months passed and then, finally, another piece of red glass came to the king. He examined it carefully, and found it indistinguishable from the Pompeii glass.

Pettenkofer? The son of the apothecary?

Oh. Nephew. That's right, nephew. Whoever he is, he's a genius.

The glass was perfect. It was exactly what Ludwig had dreamed of, and its formula had exactly the effect Ludwig had hoped. Within months the red glass of Bavaria was in demand all over Europe. It was a stunning scientific upset, and Ludwig wanted to meet this son of the apothecary . . . nephew, rather.

It was already becoming clear that while Max Pettenkofer had been born a commoner, he probably wouldn't die one.

In 1847, a favorite of the king, Pettenkofer became professor of medical chemistry at the University of Munich. His new position was a highly respected one and, what was more, carried with it an annual salary of seven hundred guldens, two measures of wheat, and seven measures of rye.

King Ludwig's career was not doing as well, however, and the sordid liaison with Lola Montez was coming to a head. In 1848, with affairs of state almost entirely in Lola's unstable hands, the nobility stepped in and forced the king to abdicate in favor of his son. Lola was banished and fled to America.

The new king, who like Max Pettenkofer had been named for Maximilian I, shared his father's eye for glass and Pettenkofer survived the overthrow, losing no influence at court.

And soon, there was more than red glass to his credit. Bavaria's cement had been inferior to that made in Portland, England. Pettenkofer invented a process that greatly improved Bavarian cement and thus equalized the competition. He also discovered a technique by which wood could be turned into a gas that could light the cities of northern Europe. Construction of a public wood gas system based on Pettenkofer's work was soon under way in the city of Basel, Switzerland.

When Uncle Franz died in 1850, King Maximilian II automatically named Pettenkofer to the post of royal apothecary. Just as automatically, Pettenkofer accepted. It increased his income, helped him keep his hand in medicine, and allowed him and Helene to move into the big house where they had spent their childhood. No one, of course, expected Max to actually mix medicines in the apothecary shop. He was involved in far, far more important matters.

The king, impressed with the accomplishments of Herr Doktor Pettenkofer, had instructed him to attract more talent to the University of Munich. Herr Doktor Pettenkofer immediately began systematically to raid the other great universities of Europe for master chemists. He even persuaded his old hero, Liebig, to join the faculty. And at the same time Max was hard at work designing a radical innovation that would later be called central heating.

It was an interesting project, insofar as it touched on the young chemist's pet theories involving the relationship between the human body and its environment. The interaction, his experiments had convinced him, was profound. Health was directly related to the availability of shelter, fresh air, clear water, and clean surroundings. Clean living meant healthful living. It was true, truer than the late John Wesley had ever guessed, that cleanliness was next to godliness.

As he had become increasingly certain of this point, he had become convinced of the absolute futility of doctors, leeches, nostrums, and salves. As any physician should be able to see, illness claimed the young, the old, the crippled, the poor . . . those in precarious health and those who lived in unhealthful (that is, filthy) surroundings. The enemy wasn't pox, typhoid, or even the cholera—it was unhygienic conditions. The solution wasn't cure—it was prevention!

He perceived this as no man before him had, and with the perception would grow a lifework and a scientific discipline. But Max's learning bridged disciplines, and his artistic yearnings had left him with a decidedly humanitarian bent. It wasn't enough to discover . . . it was necessary to act! And to act for the betterment of man!

As the first scientific hygienist, as later generations would call him, Max Pettenkofer was appalled by the terrible conditions under which most of Munich's population lived. He remembered abject poverty from his youngest days, and knew the terrible effect it had. He visited rat-infested walk-ups where whole families lived in tiny rooms that stank of human excrement. The water they drank was filthy—full, the idealistic young scientist was certain, of hundreds of unnamed poisons. No wonder the burghers wouldn't drink it! And no wonder so many of the poor, who had nothing cleaner to drink, died of fevers and diarrhea.

He pleaded their case to King Max II, who listened thoughtfully.

The water, for instance, he argued passionately . . . the city could build aqueducts into the Alpine foothills and bring fresh water to the public faucets. . . .

Expensive? Yes, Your Majesty, but . . .

And then the question of heating. The body shouldn't be allowed to grow too cold, or health would fail. The people used stoves, but they were inefficient. Sometimes their smoldering and ill-designed stoves used up all the air and entire families died. Sometimes they caused fires that raged through whole blocks. . . .

Cholera was on the move again, the travelers said. Once again it had broken out of Calcutta, and moved north and west. Max worried about it, as the other doctors did, but there was nothing he could do about cholera itself. There *was*, however, something he could do about poor hygiene. So he didn't waste his time with cholera; he thought about hygiene, and he polished his presentations to the king.

In the sense that a good king is one who listens to his advisers, King Max II was a good king. However, he didn't listen to the professor solely because he was obligated to. The simple fact was that it was almost impossible *not* to listen to him.

Max paced the floor as he argued his points and painted a picture of a better, healthier future. He emphasized his points with dramatic gestures as his voice rose and fell, growing occasionally indignant, sometimes pleading, often conspiratorial. Max had grown a fine, long moustache, which he waxed each morning and twirled expertly when he chose to. His fine mind was the basis of his insights, but his training on the stage did much to enhance his influence.

The paternity of great ideas is elusive. The king didn't exactly listen to Max's sometimes abstract thoughts. Rather, he listened to Max, allowed himself to be mesmerized by him, and the ideas, as they occurred, were the king's own. It was the king's desire to encourage science at the university, the king's desire to help his more miserable subjects. . . . Take central heating, for instance. That was

one of Maximilian's finer ideas. It was indeed fortunate
that he had such a brilliant servant as Max Pettenkofer to
carry it out.

Pettenkofer was almost wild with excitement. The project to heat the tenements of the poor automatically involved central furnaces that supplied heated air, via
ductwork, to each room. That meant he would have to
study the behavior of air and other gases in buildings, and
their relationship to health. What could be more funda-
mental to the great questions of hygiene?

One of the first things that Max had to do was devise a
way to measure air quality, something more precise than
his own nose. He knew that stinking, foul air generally
contained more carbon dioxide than pure, fresh air. He
quickly invented a method for testing for CO_2.

The poor watched Herr Professor Doktor Pettenkofer's behavior with respectful bewilderment. He arrived
in their apartments with a bottle of water, which he
promptly poured out. The bottle filled with air and the
professor poured a measure of limewater into it, capped it,
and sloshed the limewater around, sending it swirling in a
mist through the trapped air. Then he uncapped the bottle
and added a drop of chemical to the limewater, which instantly turned bright red. The scientist added more drops
until, suddenly, with no warning, the red vanished and
the limewater became clear again. The number of drops
told Max how much carbon dioxide was present in the air
of the room.

How much CO_2 was tolerable? Max wasn't precisely
sure, of course. But when he had people with bad breath
breathe into his bottle, the expired air usually had up to
ten parts per thousand of carbon dioxide. One part per
thousand sounded, to the professor, like a practical natural
limit for clean air.

Like other socially conscious scientific figures of his

time, Max gave public lectures intended to raise the understanding of the poor. Here he put on his best performances, playing to the audience, cajoling them, instructing them.

They didn't understand his chemistry, but they got the message. At the gut level, it was easy to understand. Things that smelled bad *were* bad, because they had poisons in them. Filth was the epitome of illness. Stinking miasmas rose from marshes and polluted rivers, and caused disease. Poisons flowed in discolored water. The clean life was a healthful life.

The king thought about an aqueduct to bring clean water to his subjects, and as he thought about it it became more and more his own idea. How, he asked his court genius, Max Pettenkofer, could such an aqueduct be built? How much would it cost?

It was an ambitious scheme, but the more the king thought about it, the better it seemed.

Max, in the meantime, studied the periodic table, fascinated by the precise order of the elements and their valences. How could the new knowledge be put to use? He devised a chemical method of reviving the colors in old paintings.

He used his dramatic talents to provide a series of public lectures on nutrition. The talks were aimed at workingmen. The lectures were based on reason, of course, but when Herr Professor Pettenkofer was in good form they were often more like sermons, full of cleansing fire and poisonous brimstone. Nutrition, he bellowed, was one of the keys to health. Good food, clean water, fresh air . . . that was proper hygiene, and common sense as well. What rational creature, given a choice, would eat bad food, drink stinking water, breathe foul air?

Everything that Max touched turned to scientific gold. His arguments that a city needed a supply of clean water became more and more popular, and his papers were in demand by all the major scientific journals. His name was recognized by scientists all over the world, and on the streets of Munich the common people pointed him out to their sons and daughters. The king enjoyed his company and solicited his advice on matters large and small. There was little jealousy. Munich thought of him as a doctor, not a chemist, and Bavaria had need of medical heroes.

Especially now.

Travelers were bringing news of still another cholera epidemic. It had killed thousands in Calcutta and had cropped up on the routes of the British opium traders in far-off China. Munich residents aged twenty and over still remembered, could never forget, the wave of death in 1836. Among the poor, everyone had lost a wife, a mother, a brother, a sister, a playmate. With each rumor, apprehension rippled through the city's collective psyche. Was cholera to return? If so, what was to be done?

It was natural that the king should ask Max Pettenkofer. Whom else would he ask? They thought of him as a doctor, but he was really a chemist—the scientific disciplines had not yet separated, at least in the minds of kings and commoners, and they looked at Max in admiration, hope, and anticipation. But for once, the court's apothecary and scientific magician was at a loss for an answer.

Thoughtfully, Max sifted the rumors, talked to doctors who had seen the results of the last epidemic, and combed the scientific literature. He pushed his mind, trying to bring the precise chemical reactions he knew to bear on the subject.

One thing was immediately evident. Cholera wasn't a contagion. It didn't pass from person to person, engulfing whole households the way smallpox did. It seemed to have a preference for the young, the old, and the weak, but it struck the healthy as well. It killed a father and didn't touch the mother; it killed a grandmother and let her husband live; it killed a child and didn't touch its siblings. The poor, presumably because of their wretched living conditions and resultant poor hygiene, were the most susceptible—but many of them escaped.

That conclusion was a popular one among the upper classes, insofar as what he said was exactly what the king wanted to hear. There was always a tendency for the population to flee a city struck by cholera, interrupting trade and closing down factories. If the people could only be made to understand that cholera wasn't contagious, there would be less panic and, as a result, less economic damage.

As the years passed, the rumors of cholera came more frequently. They crossed the desert with the caravans and traveled through the vastness of Russia with pilgrims and gypsy storytellers. In Calcutta, funeral pyres licked at the sky. Death crept through Siam. Bloated, blackened bodies drifted down the rivers of China, tumbling over and over as the fishes fed. Pilgrims in Mecca collapsed and died. Cholera seized the Ottoman Empire.

Herr Professor Doktor Max Pettenkofer listened thoughtfully to the stories, turning the puzzle over and over in his mind, applying the powers of reason that had produced Pompeii glass, wood gas, and an improved cement.

He started, as he always did, with principles he knew and trusted, the precise processes of chemistry.

Disease was, as every educated person knew, generally caused by poisonous miasmas, bad airs, dank and stinking airs, rotten airs, airs of death. The malnourished poor, surrounded by filth and weakened by the ravages of more common diseases, were naturally the most affected by the poison. The more Max thought about it, the more he became convinced that cholera might best be fought by an improvement in the living conditions of the poor.

And yet, as to precisely what caused it, he had no theories.

Cholera now was in Russia. A million people had died there, travelers said. Max intensified his efforts to improve conditions in the slums. The healthier the people were, the more easily they could resist all diseases, including cholera.

It was in the Mediterranean now. Spain.

In a far-off South American port, a British survey ship, the HMS *Beagle*, was denied permission to land. The city fathers had heard rumors of cholera in London. Frustrated, a young naturalist named Charles Darwin paced the decks, miserable at being denied the opportunity to collect local insects, plants, and animals.

Eighteen fifty passed. Then 1851, 1852, 1853. Paris, Hamburg, Berlin. Munich waited, terrified.

But again the wave of death seemed to break around the city and to pass it by. Cholera was in London, New York, Glasgow, and Madrid. Optimists in Munich expressed the hopeful opinion that, this time, their city really would be spared.

But the optimism was just that. In the summer of 1854, the year that Pettenkofer turned thirty-six, the wave of death broke backward and cholera spread through Munich. Again the windows of the palace were closed, despite the oppressive heat. Carts carried the bodies through the streets. Max's apprentices mixed bouquets of herbs and spices to protect the royal noses from the bad air. King Max appointed a commission to deal with the epidemic, a group that naturally included the most famous physician and surgeon of all, Professor Pettenkofer.

The scientist still had no answers, but he had a prejudice that with cholera, as with everything else he had tackled, the environment had to be the critical factor. That was the lesson of his lifework.

So, assuming cholera was caused by some environmental factor, what would that factor be? Probably, he reasoned, a poison.

Pettenkofer's first action was to requisition a copy of the most accurate map of the city, that drawn up by the Army's defense group. Using the Army maps he recorded the geographic location of each victim's home.

As the pestilence raged he sat before the maps, pondering, pushing his mind to see the pattern that, he knew, should be there. Finally, as the cholera epidemic reached its peak, his patience was rewarded. Specific areas of the city, relatively small areas in fact, seemed to account for most of the mortality.

On the maps, Max drew bold lines in red ink around the districts of death. Areas that had just a smattering of cases were enclosed in green. Blue lines marked off the sectors in which cholera was rare.

By now it was autumn, and the disease had begun to fade from the city. Max had been able to offer no help this time, but now he had, he reckoned, the clues he needed. He would study those clues and from them he would find the answer. The next time, he assured the king, it would be different.

He studied the maps and visited the neighborhoods involved. What were the differences between them? The hardest-hit sectors were poor ones, of course. He had expected that, but it wasn't the complete answer. There were other poverty areas that had escaped almost entirely.

Why?

It had to be some critical difference in the environment. But what?

Patiently, the scientist sorted through his data, arranging and rearranging it, worrying at it, looking for patterns. He had faith in the scientific method, and patience, and he knew he would eventually find the answer. Finally, as he always knew it would, it came to him in a rush of insight.

The hardest-hit neighborhoods were all in low-lying, almost marshy areas. Something was different, indeed. Something very critical to the environment.

Soil condition!

The cholera areas were in low-lying areas near the river, just exactly where a thinking man would expect miasmas to form. The earth in such places seemed unusually porous, which would allow the passage of air into and out of the soil. The air seemed dank and, in the wetter areas where there were a lot of rotting plants, fetid.

The answer had eluded him for so long, but now that he saw it in the right perspective, why . . . it had been obvious all along! The chemistry was all there! The soil contained material that could rot when exposed to water and air. The material in the soil was probably activated in some way, to produce a miasma . . . the same way, in principle, as hydrochloric acid activated sodium sulfide to produce the smell of rotten eggs. Swamps were notorious for spawning many diseases, including malaria. Why not cholera as well?

Max hired workmen to plant pipes in the ground at various locations in the red-, blue-, and green-lined areas. He recorded how fast the pipes filled with water, and the level the water reached. The results confirmed his suspicion. Cholera was chiefly confined to locations where the water table was high and where the soil was loose.

Air, he explained to the king, could easily pass through soil. As a demonstration he placed a small bird in a flask and packed the neck of the flask with loose dirt. The king watched intently, waiting for the bird to suffocate. But it didn't. Herr Professor Doktor Pettenkofer was, once again, correct.

So, Pettenkofer continued, the clean air went into the damp soil and there it activated a chemical reaction that resulted in a terrible poison. People who lived nearby were likely to get cholera. People who lived on the hills, where the soil was rocky and the breeze swept away what poisons were produced, rarely became ill with cholera.

The solution bolstered Max's broader health theories. Cholera, like most other diseases, could be fought with better hygiene. The poor needed ventilation so that the poisons wouldn't collect in their living spaces. They needed sunlight and a proper diet so that they could resist what poisons they were exposed to.

Also, when the aqueduct was finally completed—which would be soon now—the water would be better and that would probably help, too. As everyone knew, Professor Pettenkofer was a vocal advocate of fresh water.

But at the same time he despised narrow-minded scientists who claimed that cholera was this one thing, or that one thing. The miasmas themselves resulted from a combination of factors in the soil and the air, and health itself was a relationship between the strength of body chemistry and the potency of poisons in the air, water, and food. Health was environment, and the environment was a relationship among all things. It wasn't, as one English know-nothing was now claiming, water alone.

The fellow's name was Snow, John Snow. The events upon which he based his simplistic claim were purported to have occurred in London in 1849, at the height of England's epidemic, but it wasn't published until 1854, five years later. Max Pettenkofer read the paper carefully, though with some amusement.

The man had apparently done the same sort of geographic studies that he, Max Pettenkofer, had done. In that, Snow obviously had good instincts . . . but little insight. He had failed entirely to consider the soil and the water table, jumping instead to the absurd conclusion that cholera was a contagion carried in the water. If it was contagious, why didn't everyone get it? Snow had apparently failed to ask himself the question, and had jumped to the overly simplistic conclusion that cholera was caused by one factor, not many.

Unlike Munich, which was served by water wells, London had two public water companies. Carried away by speculation, Snow presented a poorly reasoned argument that cholera was carried by the water supplied by one of those companies. Why, the man even claimed to have stopped one local epidemic by removing the handle of the pump on Broad Street, which was at the center of the cholera-ridden area.

Oversimplification. Oversimplification and hubris. Who did Snow think he was? Max Pettenkofer, for one, had never heard of him. But, unfortunately, the public didn't appreciate the complexity of the issue, and many people were impressed with the Englishman's ideas.

Occasionally one of the aristocrats, usually someone who should have known better, would make the mistake of asking Max about Snow's claim and the Broad Street pump.

Professor Pettenkofer was always ready with the facts, and the fact was that the particular epidemic Snow claimed to have stopped was already tapering off at the time he claimed to have stopped it. It had hit its peak on September 2, with 125 new cases. On subsequent days it fell rapidly to 58, then 52, then 28, then 22, and then, the day before the famous pump handle was removed, 14.

Pettenkofer twirled his moustache and smiled. Obviously some environmental condition had naturally righted itself and the disease was already on the decline before Snow stepped in. The British scientist—if you wanted to call him a scientist—could have achieved the same results with chants and incantations. All in all, the Snow paper was a gross misinterpretation of the facts.

Those who inquired, including the king, didn't question Max Pettenkofer's judgment in the matter. Who were

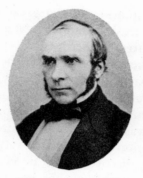

DR. JOHN SNOW

Courtesy National Library of Medicine

they, after all, to second-guess a genius? He said, and they believed, that cholera was related to the environment, to the condition of the soil and the consequent foul particles or poisons in the air.

But why did the miasmas come in some years and not in others?

Max explained that the critical elements were the soil, the groundwater level, and the amount of decaying matter trapped in the interstices between the soil particles.

The miasma itself came from, or was activated by, rotting plant debris in the soil. If the soil was high and rocky, there was little plant matter in it to produce miasmas. There was plenty of plant matter in low-lying land, but in most years the air couldn't penetrate far enough into swampy ground to be affected, since the soil was waterlogged. But in certain impossible-to-predict years when the summer was especially dry, the air could penetrate the swampy ground to unusual depths and start the reaction that ultimately produced the cholera miasma. Max had figures to prove that Munich's groundwater level was unusually low in the summers of 1836 and 1854—peak years for cholera.

As the second cholera epidemic faded into memory,

Max turned his attention to the great viaduct that, one
day, would bring fresh mountain water to the citizens of
Munich. He lectured, experimented, theorized, and explained. He worked diligently for the improvement of
hygiene in the poor sections of the city.

Civilization advanced in other disciplines, as well. Sam-
uel Colt revolutionized the manufacture of small arms.
The plaster cast was invented by a Dutch Army surgeon.
The word "evolution" was coined. Rayon was invented.
Victoria Falls was discovered by the intrepid Livingstone.
Matthew Maury published his monumental work *The
Physical Geography of the Sea*. A German botanist, Nathan-
ael Pringsheim, used a microscope to observe, for the first
time, sperm entering the ovum in plants. In 1857 a
Frenchman named Pasteur demonstrated that the process
of fermentation couldn't take place in a sterile environ-
ment.

Pettenkofer, intent on other matters, paid no notice to
Pasteur. Pasteur was interested in beer making and Max
was not particularly interested in the brewmaster's craft
or, for that matter, in beer. Pettenkofer was disgusted by
the ravages of drunkenness he saw around him, and he,
personally, didn't touch the stuff.

Again the cholera rose up out of India and was reported
in Russia. Then Turkey, then Egypt. London. Again the
poor followed the body carts through the streets of Munich,
lamenting the suddenly dead.

It wasn't contagious, Pettenkofer reassured the city fathers. There was a solution, but the solution was the general improvement of public health. The healthier the
public was, the less cholera there would be. And not only
cholera, but other diseases as well. Even typhoid.

The epidemic peaked and declined.

In the meantime Pettenkofer's dream of public health
had caught fire, and the great campaign spread to other

cities. The cry was to banish foul air, bad food, and filth. Cleanliness was next to godliness.

The public health crusade was a broadly based movement with roots in aesthetics as well as the sciences. Europeans and even the Americans were realizing that their cities smelled bad and they perceived that somehow, in a way that transcended even the disease-bearing miasmas, the stench was a statement about the living conditions that bred it.

Karl Marx, struggling to understand the poverty he saw, blamed environment even for the animalistic and often criminal behavior of the poor. "It is not the consciousness of men that determines their existence," he wrote; ". . . their social existence determines their consciousness."

But Max Pettenkofer, as a scientist, was the one who could quantify the thoughts and speak of bettering the poor in terms of concrete goals. Clean water. Fresh air. Warmth in the winter. Adequate and proper diets.

Progress in conservative Bavaria was frustratingly slow and Munich, as it always had, lagged behind the public health efforts of London. This was maddening to Pettenkofer, who was foremost in the scientific study of man's immediate environment. Was it not Pettenkofer in Munich who had showed so precisely that the human excretion was made up of many chemicals, and that those chemicals were related to the intake of food, water, and air? Was it not Pettenkofer in Munich who had studied the effects of malnutrition on the body? Was it not Pettenkofer in Munich who was in the best position to show, with hard, inarguable numbers, that filth spread disease and that a slum was a danger to an entire city? It was!

But it was Snow and other hygienists in London who had first persuaded the city fathers to install running water in individual apartments and to construct sewer connections to each house. And it was in London that the death rate fell from forty per thousand to twenty-two per thousand. Pettenkofer's beloved Munich, though cleaner than before, couldn't compare to London.

Pettenkofer saw this backwardness as a shame on his city, and he argued all the harder. He used all the theatrics at his command; he used all the logic; he appealed to the burghers' sense of social responsibility. But their loyalty, always, was to their pocketbooks.

Not that he didn't get results. He did. In 1865, the great aqueduct was finished and the sparkling Alpine water flowed freely from the public taps. The incidence of typhoid fell immediately and the health of the city generally improved.

The aqueduct was a magnificent accomplishment and a first great step toward public health, but Herr Professor Doktor Pettenkofer was far from satisfied. It wouldn't do to stop there, he cautioned. The water must be piped to every house. There must be adequate ventilation. Food must improve. Sewers and toilets must be installed.

Though Munich lagged behind London in matters of public health, Max Pettenkofer, by age forty-eight, lagged behind no one. He was a Renaissance man, perhaps the most prestigious scientist in Europe. His arguments, always backed up by experimental data, carried an enormous impact in areas as diverse as public health and industrial chemistry, and, thanks to his work on cholera, he was the greatest of all the miasmatists.

Not that the cholera work had no skeptics. There are always skeptics. A certain Professor Drasche, of Vienna, claimed that there was an outbreak of cholera near Krain, in the Karst Mountains of Croatia, where the soil was rocky. How, in accordance with the Pettenkofer theory, could miasmas form from rocky soil?

Challenged, Max immediately traveled to Krain and be-

gan an exhaustive study of the outbreak at issue. As before, he mapped the homes of the victims and keyed his
maps to the soil conditions. It was true . . . the soil *did*
seem rocky to the untrained eye. But, Max pointed out,
the rocky subsoil was rent with fractures. That was probably what allowed the air to get in and the miasmas to
form.

Vindicated, he returned to Munich to sit with kings,
ministers, and financiers, discussing hygiene in the slums,
arguing for better food for the poor, extolling the virtues
of cleanliness and adequate ventilation. Everywhere the
great miasmatist went, he received a respectful hearing.

But the matter of cholera wouldn't rest. There were reports, respectful but at the same time impertinent, that
cholera epidemics in Gibraltar and Malta hadn't followed
the pattern the miasma theory dictated. Again, the reports
said, the soil conditions had been wrong, but cholera had
occurred anyway.

Max could have ignored the reports, certain as he was
that they were based on misunderstanding and misinterpretation . . . but to ignore them might signify a weakness of confidence, a fear. Besides, he was a scientist and
the truth needed defending. He selected the best of his
assistants, packed his equipment, and boarded a train.

He had been right all along, of course. In Gibraltar
much of the soil near the red areas on his map was quite
porous. There were outbreaks in high, rockier locations
. . . but, as at Krain, a trained eye could spot breaks and
fractures in the surface. That was obviously how the air
got into the soil and how the miasmas got out.

Also, he learned to his satisfaction, records taken from
the area's two hundred wells showed that, just prior to the
epidemic, there had been a marked rise in the groundwater level, followed by an abrupt decline.

As for Malta, yes, it was rocky. But the sandstone surfaces were soft and porous. He could cut them with a knife. Air, then, could enter the rock itself!

It was, he reasoned . . . sort of a stony swamp.

Some scientists still seemed dissatisfied, however, and there was talk that Pettenkofer's arguments were growing somehow strained. Pettenkofer ignored the doubters. It astonished and disheartened him to consider how few keen observers there seemed to be in science these days.

Back in Munich, he concentrated on measuring the input and output of animals. He kept them in glass jars, measuring how much air, food, and water they consumed, weighing and analyzing their urine and feces. Even in his fifties he worked feverishly, certain that the interaction between man and his environment could be described in precise chemical formulas. Each day brought a new success and buoyed his sense of impending discovery.

It was, like the year of his birth, a time of change. King Max II died and was replaced on the throne by King Ludwig II, a handsome, romantic man who displayed a charming eccentricity. As the 1860s ended the loose confederation of Germanic kingdoms that included Bavaria found itself locked in a great war with France and, through the process of war, was then brought under German rule by the Iron Chancellor, Otto von Bismarck. Across the Atlantic, Alexander Graham Bell invented the telephone. James Clerk Maxwell published a paper announcing that electricity and magnetism were different manifestations of the same thing.

In Prussia, Robert Koch, a diminutive country doctor with heavy spectacles, received a microscope as a present from his wife. He kissed her and then, in a boyish display of impatience, set the toy up on the windowsill where he could catch the sunlight in its mirror. She watched, lovingly and indulgently, as he peered through it. Men, she had learned long ago, never completely grow up.

In Munich, Max Pettenkofer sat with King Ludwig and

talked about the concept of public sewers. The king listened intently. The professor was fluent, and knowledgeable on almost every facet of human endeavor.

At night, or whenever he had a spare moment, Max leafed through the journals.

Koch? From Prussia?

Max looked at the name on the paper and searched his memory. Koch. Koch. Never heard of him.

Quickly, the great miasmatist scanned the report. Koch, whoever he was, had identified tiny red rods swimming in the blood of cattle that had died of anthrax. He had used sterile slivers of wood to transfer these beasties to the bloodstreams of mice, and the mice, too, had died of anthrax.

Interesting. Probably meaningless.

The professor turned the page.

Life was busy and, at the same time, luxurious. Max's daughter and two sons were grown now and, while he missed the childish voices in the house, he had more time for work. Increasingly, his days were spent lecturing and explaining, to audiences as varied as paupers and kings. The years passed. He collected award after award. In the winter, the whitecapped Alps glittered beautifully in the sun. In the summer he walked beneath the spreading horse chestnut trees, taking in the air and thinking about the new science of hygiene.

It was a science that, to be successful, had to have an almost unheard-of degree of public support. The burghers were right. It would cost a lot of money.

Money.

What was the worth of health?

Facing that question with the precision of a chemist and the passion of a sociologist, he composed two public lectures to make his point. They were first delivered in 1873, to audiences of laymen.

Why, he asked, appealing to their patriotic inclinations,

do English cities have a lower death rate than German ones? Do the English have a better climate?

He paused, to let the audience consider the notoriously cold and drizzly British weather. Pettenkofer always liked to get a chuckle. It brought him closer to the audience.

Do the British have a better geographic situation? Do they have a firmer national character? Are English doctors, perchance, better trained than German ones? Are they more skillful? Are their pharmacies better? Are their hospitals superior? Are there fewer swindlers selling patent medicines and other quackeries, or fewer idiots to buy them?

Or is their sounder public health a credit to better nutrition, housing, clothing, labor and occupations, customs and habits, legislation, or social conditions? Is it the result of better sewerage and water supplies?

He appealed to his countrymen's aesthetic sense. Can something that smells foul, or tastes foul, be healthy? Can human excrement, dumped to molder in the gutters, be good for passersby? Pleasant things are healthy things, and the poor, if only they were surrounded by a more pleasant environment, would be healthier.

But, of course, the poor can't pay for any of these things. . . .

He appealed to the audience's humanity.

"In every large community," he said, "there are always many people who have not the means to procure for themselves the things that are absolutely necessary to a healthy life. Those who have more than they need must contribute to supply these wants in their own interest. If the dwellings of the poor become infected with typhoid and cholera, that is the threat to the health of the richest people, also. A city must consider itself a family, so to say. Care must be taken of everybody in the house, [including] those who do not or cannot contribute toward its support."

But, most of all, he appealed to the pocketbook.

When a laborer is sick, he doesn't work. But his wife and children still eat. When a disease like typhoid or cholera sweeps through the tenements, the factories produce less. Machinery, purchased at great cost, sits idle. If the laborer dies his dependents inevitably, and through whatever means, become public charges.

Yes, it will cost money to improve the public health. It will cost money, but it will save more. If Munich could reach a death rate as low as London's, the public coffers would ultimately save 25 million guldens a year.

And that touched a chord in Munich. Pettenkofer's arguments were compelling and his performance was powerful. There was a large investment involved, certainly. A huge investment. But the investment would be repaid, again and again. If the poor would benefit as well, that was all to the good.

In 1879 the city established the Hygienic Institute, the world's first major laboratory for the scientific study of hygiene. From all over the world, Pettenkofer received applications from young scientists who wanted to study under him at the institute. He chose the best. Pettenkofer had always been a prolific writer, but now his production of scientific papers intensified even more.

Koch? He kept hearing the name Koch. Who was he? A backcountry doctor?

Engrossed in his own studies on man and his environment, Pettenkofer hardly noticed when, the same year that the Hygienic Institute opened, the bacterium responsible for gonorrhea was found. The following year typhoid was linked with a microbe. The malarial parasite swam into microscopic focus for the first time in 1881.

Pettenkofer studied ventilation, nutrition, and poisons in the environment.

And then, a distraction.

Koch again?

What did he mean, no soil factor was needed to explain cholera? That was idiotic! If cholera was communicable, everybody who was exposed would get it. They didn't. End of argument.

True enough, Pettenkofer conceded, the morbid particle in the miasma might be a creature of some sort . . . but there was more involved than just that. Just as it took hydrochloric acid to turn sodium sulfide into the rotten-smelling hydrogen sulfide gas, it took an activating factor to turn the air into cholera miasma.

Still, Koch's arguments appealed to the masses. That frustrated Max, but he reasoned that he was faced with more a problem in communication than an enigma of science. The environment was so complicated that the human mind rebelled. That was why Snow, for instance, claimed public health was a matter of clean water and public sewers. He was right enough, as far as he went, but he overlooked nutrition and ventilation. It was easy to explain cholera by postulating some theoretical microbe. It was easy, but it was wrong.

Pettenkofer groped for a way to explain it to his students.

Say there was some factor in the air, some factor x. Perhaps the factor x was one of Koch's beasties. All right. You've got factor x in the air, but it can't cause disease. Not by itself. There must be something else in the soil, some factor . . . call it y. Y, by itself, won't make you sick either.

But if x gets into the soil and unites with y, then . . . you get something quite different, call it z, some poison, some miasma. Z causes cholera.

X plus y equals z!

What could be simpler?

Another year passed. It was 1882.

Koch again!

He did what?

Tuberculosis?

Tuberculosis was a dread disease and it was known to be contagious. Yet Koch had dared to experiment with it and to isolate some tiny beaded rods that, if you believed Koch, caused it.

If. If. If you believed Koch.

Max was skeptical, as a scientist should be, but the public wasn't, and neither was it in the mood to listen to the complicated mutterings of an old Bavarian professor. Koch had dared to work with tuberculosis and had pulled it off! What a brave man he must be!

Koch was a hero, the talk of Berlin. With the Germanys united, Munich was a backwater, a city to visit if you wished to see the past.

Max buried himself in work and tried to ignore the growing powers of the only rival he had ever known, but it was impossible. There were cholera rumors again, from India, and Koch turned his attention to the problem.

The problem? What problem, Pettenkofer wanted to know. The problem had already been solved!

Max was outraged when Koch stated cavalierly that the soils in Bombay and Genoa, where cholera had occurred, didn't meet the Pettenkofer specifications. The microbiologist claimed the soil was hard and compact, and impervious to air. Koch was as stubbornly, maliciously wrong as John Snow had been. It was almost a public treachery, a scientist preaching that cholera was communicable! How was the population going to react to that, if the disease came again?

Exasperated, Pettenkofer set aside his more important public-health projects and turned his attention to the tiresome business of proving himself correct still another time. He commissioned an Italian engineer to survey the soils in the areas that Koch had talked about. Pettenkofer paid the engineer handsomely, and the engineer, who was no fool, found exactly what his patron had paid him to find—foul and porous soils.

Koch, Pettenkofer said, must have used poor maps.

The scientists and nobility listened respectfully to Herr Professor Doktor Pettenkofer, but there was a different quality to their stares now. They seemed distant, speculative.

They liked Koch.

Imagine the courage, to *actually go seeking the microbe that caused tuberculosis!* Of such acts are heroes made.

But Pettenkofer laughed. A cholera bacterium? Will Koch never quit speculating beyond his data? The man hadn't claimed to have actually *found* that cholera beastie of his, had he?

No?

Max had thought not.

Why was it so difficult for them to understand? It was very simple, really. If the soil was wet but not so wet as to

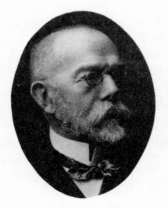

DR. ROBERT KOCH
Courtesy National Library of Medicine

be waterlogged, and if air could get in, and if there was rotten plant material in the soil . . . then, and only then, you had a miasma.

Munich was a beautiful place to live. In the spring the breezes were balmy and the boughs of the horse chestnut trees whispered overhead. Music, the best music of the ages, floated over the city. Life was pleasant, thanks to the great hygienist, Herr Professor Doktor Max Pettenkofer. Young men automatically tipped their hats to him now. Young women curtsied.

But in Berlin, Max heard, they lined the streets to see the hero Koch pass by.

Again King Cholera rose in India, and the funeral pyres lighted the banks of the Ganges.

Medical scientists in Europe had learned by now to watch the disease more closely, and to monitor and document its spread. Pilgrims brought it to Mecca, and from there it jumped in 1883 to a town at the Mediterranean terminus of the new Suez Canal, where a festival was in progress. Within half a week the death toll there had reached a hundred a day, and the festival-goers had fled to their home villages in panic. Death followed them. Thousands died in Cairo.

The Europeans watched the developing epidemic uneasily but, to the new generation of microbiologists, the recurrence of cholera represented a sterling opportunity. The theories were in place: If you listened to Koch, which almost everyone did, there was a bacterium responsible. There had to be.

In Berlin, a plan circulated to send a commission to the stricken areas to isolate the bacterium and then study it, before it moved farther. Koch, of course, was named to head the expedition. Pettenkofer wasn't mentioned.

There was more involved, however, than a mere epidemic that threatened the poor of Europe. A nationalistic rivalry had developed between Koch's followers in Germany and Pasteur's students in France, Germany's ancient archenemy. France, too, would send an expedition.

Both groups landed at Alexandria within days of one another, in August of 1883, and set up their equipment.

The two teams, reflecting the biases of Pasteur and Koch, proceeded differently. The French took blood and feces from the sick and attempted to transfer the disease by means of inoculation to rats, mice, guinea pigs, and other small animals. This strategy, however, produced no results and, in early September, one of the French scientists contracted cholera and died. His death so unnerved his colleagues that, a short time later, they decamped and fled back to Paris.

Koch's group remained and continued their effort to search with microscopes for the cholera bacteria. Finally, Koch stared triumphantly down the barrel of his instrument at a tiny, odd-looking creature that, because of its tail, reminded him of a comma.

It was a short, curved rod. It was very small . . . only a fifth as long as a red blood cell was wide. It moved beneath the microscope, driven through the liquid by its whipping tail. The beastie was found in twelve patients and ten corpses.

Ever cautious, Koch wanted to observe further but the Egyptian epidemic was on the wane, so he took his party on to India, to the spawning ground itself. The scientists worked into the winter and by February Koch was satisfied. There was no doubt. Cholera was caused by the comma-shaped organism.

Word of the success traveled quickly to Germany. Koch had succeeded again! And he had beaten the French!

Pettenkofer groused.

Fools!

Of course, Koch had found an organism. What could you expect of a man like Koch, a supposed scientist who routinely ignored the facts? Microbe or no microbe, cholera depended on local soil conditions, as any idiot who looked at the data could see. The location was all important.

Koch arrived back in Berlin on May 2, 1884, and received the kind of welcome reserved for heroes. Patriotism in the newly forged land of Germany ran high, and Koch had done more than just confirm his earlier findings. He had demonstrated the superiority of German science over that of the loathed French and, for that matter, the fumbling British. In Berlin, the kaiser hung a medal around Koch's neck and the Reichstag awarded him 100,000 marks. Beautiful ladies waited to dance with him at a court reception.

In Munich, sixty-six-year-old Max fumed and raged.

Koch wasn't even a gentleman!

What did the man mean, referring to Herr Professor Doktor Max Pettenkofer so condescendingly as "Herr Localist"?

Koch wasn't only a fool, he was a disrespectful lout to boot!

Though he was outraged, Pettenkofer forced himself to continue his work in hygiene. Summer came, followed by winter, followed by spring. More and more people came to hear the great professor extol the virtues of cleanliness, nutrition, ventilation, and sanitation. Pasteur reported the production of rabies vaccine. An Englishman, Sir Charles Parsons, invented the first practical steam engine. George Eastman began the manufacture of photographic paper.

In the meantime the wave of cholera that Koch had studied in Egypt moved on in 1884 into France, Italy, and Spain. It lingered, summer after summer, killing eighty thousand Frenchmen and like numbers of Italians and Spaniards. But it didn't travel north to Pettenkofer's Germany.

Instead the wave appeared to weaken and die out. As

the 1880s ended it looked as though, this time, Germany would indeed be spared.

Then the disease struck again in Persia and Afghanistan and, thanks to increasingly modern transportation, exploded north into the heart of Russia that same summer. It was in Baku, in St. Petersburg, in Moscow. A million died. The disease accompanied the refugees west.

Eighteen ninety-two. Hamburg.

First there was one case, in the most squalid part of the city. Then there was a second. A fifth. A hundredth. Residents, understanding Koch's point that cholera was contagious, fled the city. Schools closed. Funeral processions wound toward the churchyards.

The German government resolved to send a commission to Hamburg and, again, Pettenkofer was ignored. Koch was chosen instead.

Koch soon reported that the cholera outbreak was clearly linked to the water. Central Hamburg was supplied by one water system and adjacent Altona and Wandsbek by others, and where the central supply stopped, so did cholera. The demarcation line was sharp and clear, often running down the center of streets. John Snow, those many years before, had been correct.

The report exploded in Max Pettenkofer's mind like the recurrence of an old, old nightmare. Why did they continually make the same mistakes? Would they never learn? Any correlation with water systems was purely coincidence! Cholera depended on local soil conditions!

Koch dismissed Pettenkofer's complaints out of hand, patronizing the elderly Herr Localist down in Munich. The whole miasma theory, as far as Koch was concerned, was composed of newts' eyes, old wives' tales, and balderdash. After all, weren't the sky, sun, wind, and rain evenly allotted all across central and suburban Hamburg? Miasmas knew no boundaries, but cholera did. Cholera's boundaries, in Hamburg, corresponded exactly with the edges of the central water district.

Clearly, Koch said, the rantings of Herr Professor Doktor Pettenkofer notwithstanding, cholera was caused by a germ, one germ, and nothing else. It was communicable and it traveled in a contaminated water supply.

Pettenkofer, the grand old man of public health, was now seventy-four. He had been patient, first with Snow and later with Koch. He had been forebearing, forgiving, thick-skinned.

But now, he had had enough. Pettenkofer would solve this problem once and for all.

Koch's germ alone, he told his students still another time, wouldn't cause cholera. It wouldn't cause cholera any more than sodium sulfide would produce the smell of rotten eggs without the addition of hydrochloric acid.

He wrote to Koch, demanding to be sent a vial of the so-called comma bacillus. The purpose? So that Pettenkofer could perform a "crucial experiment" in which he would demonstrate the harmlessness of the comma creatures. Specifically, he would drink them.

In Berlin a few days later Koch stared at the letter, at first in disbelief and then with resignation. If he denied the request, Pettenkofer would surely accuse him of cowardice. But if he sent the bacteria . . .

On the other hand, was it his function to protect the doddering Herr Doktor from himself? No!

He sent a flask of bacteria cultured from a patient dying of cholera. Pettenkofer waited for it at the Hygiene Institute. When it arrived, he examined it with satisfaction. There were, he reckoned, a billion bacteria there.

Never one to ignore the drama of the moment, Herr Professor Doktor Max Pettenkofer summoned his favorite students. When they were settled and quiet in the auditorium, he told them he had a short speech to make. He made certain his words would be accurately written down.

"Even if I be mistaken and this experiment that I am making imperils my life, I shall look death quietly in the face, for what I am doing is no frivolous or cowardly act of suicide, but I shall die in the service of science as a soldier perishes on the field of honor."

He paused for effect, looking around him. The look on the young men's faces was one of rapt attention.

"Health and life," he continued, "are doubtless worldly possessions of enormous value, but they are not the most valuable of human goods. Man, who wants to occupy a higher position than the beasts, must be ready to sacrifice even life and health on behalf of higher and more ideal goods!"

Perhaps then the old scientist held the flask above him, as Goethe's Brackenburg had held the flask of poison. Then, with none of Brackenburg's hesitation, he put the container to his lips and drank. Carefully, he set the empty flask down, wiped his lips, smiled at his students, and returned to his laboratory. His students, too, went back to work . . . but they kept a close watch on their master, just in case.

The day passed and nothing happened. The next day, Pettenkofer worked contentedly in his laboratory, showing no ill effects. The next day as well he was unharmed.

Pettenkofer waited until there could be no doubt, then composed a second letter to Koch. He thanked the Berlin scientist for the cholera germs and reported that he had consumed the entire portion and was pleased to inform Herr Doktor Koch that he was in his usual good health.

Pettenkofer, pleased with himself for having demonstrated the shallowness of Koch's theory once and for all, wasn't prepared for his rival's response.

What Koch did was . . . nothing.

*   *   *

Koch and Pasteur, and their generation of microbiologists, had spent years methodically collecting evidence that diseases were caused by tiny creatures that invaded the body and poisoned it with their excretions. One demonstration, no matter how heroic (or foolish), was simply not enough to invalidate the amassed evidence.

Why didn't Pettenkofer sicken and die? The students of the new microbiology asked the question and wondered. Perhaps he was simply too old, too stubborn, too . . . perhaps . . . There was an inkling . . . not quite a hint even, yet, but an inkling. . . . Some people, intimately associated with a disease, might become somehow resistant . . . sort of . . . immune. . . .

If that was the case, Pettenkofer was simply lucky. Luckier than Daniel Carrión had been, luckier than others who would come later.

In any event, Pettenkofer's experiment posed the kind of enigma that made the new biologists scratch their heads, but it wasn't enough to make them change their minds.

In Munich, Pettenkofer's self-satisfaction turned, as the weeks and months passed, to incredulity. These men called themselves scientists, and yet they ignored his irrefutable findings!

And there was absolutely nothing he could do about it.

Max Pettenkofer's x plus y equals z theory of cholera didn't die a sudden death. Older scientists, reared in the tradition of miasma-caused disease, continued to be loyal to him, but as the years passed they died. Only in Pettenkofer's native city of Munich was there a stronghold of disciples.

Pettenkofer himself, though now of advanced age, didn't fade away either. His experiments, which were to put the hygiene movement on a scientific footing, proceeded satisfactorily. His institute grew and prospered and

in Munich, thanks to the institute, the death rate continued to fall. In 1898, the year Max turned 80, it stood at
24.7 deaths per 1,000 citizens—only 2.7 away from his
goal of equaling London.

If his ideas concerning cholera played to an empty
house, his accomplishments in hygiene enjoyed a full one.
In the area of cholera he was a reactionary force, an old
man who clung desperately to old ideas, a man who stood
against progress . . . who countered careful experiment
with theatrical gesture. But in the field of hygiene, it was
different. In hygiene, he was the true scientist, the inno-
vator.

Students continued to undergo great hardship for the
privilege of studying under the great Pettenkofer. His
name appeared again and again in the journals.

A grateful nation granted him hereditary nobility, and
the poor country boy was now introduced as His Excellency. He was no longer Max Pettenkofer, but Max von
Pettenkofer. The British Institute of Public Health gave
him a gold medal. His work on atomic weights earned him
another gold medal from the German Chemical Society.
The grateful city of Munich bestowed still another one.
He was the father of public health, and they were grateful
to him for that.

But mostly the seasons passed, and the work went on
and on and on, and Pettenkofer grew older and older. His
wife died, as did his last surviving child. In loneliness,
beset by the pains of his advanced age, he found the honors held little satisfaction.

Each one had, pointedly it seemed to him, overlooked
his greatest and most insightful contribution to mankind,
the x-plus-y-equals-z theory of cholera, a theory he had
risked his life to prove. There was no gold medal for
courage.

But he never faltered. Though he grew older he mustered his declining energies to defend the miasma theory against the onrushing tide of bacteriologists. He stood firmly and bravely against the relentless flood, but it washed around him and went on.

A perception dawned that the chemistry of proteins and bacteria was somehow infinitely more complex than the chemistry of sodium sulfide and hydrochloric acid. Biochemistry required a new way of looking at things, an imprecise way that offended the intellects of pure chemists. The study of life chemistry was budding off from its parent and becoming a separate discipline. The age of the Renaissance man was giving way to the impersonal age of specialization.

Another German, Albert Einstein, was growing up. So was Alexander Fleming, who would discover penicillin. A patent was let on the first machine gun. The first Ford rolled off the assembly line. A microbe was linked to malaria. Koch developed an inoculation for anthrax.

As His Excellency Herr Professor Doktor Max von Pettenkofer grew older and older, and didn't die, he grew increasingly bitter. It would have been better, perhaps, if the comma-shaped organisms had killed him. But fate denied him the gift of death, then and now, and he lived on.

The century turned. Radon was discovered. Max Planck formulated the quantum theory. Sigmund Freud published *The Interpretation of Dreams*. The first Zeppelin lifted into the air. Browning began manufacturing revolvers.

It was 1901. X plus y equaled z, as it always had, but nobody listened.

The revolver was cold, like the grave, like the new age that cared nothing for truth or honor or respect. The bullets nestled in their chambers.

Max von Pettenkofer caressed the metal with liver-spotted hands. The gun was heavy. He put the muzzle to his temple. This time there was no audience.

The shot echoed off the walls and down the hall. The last of the great miasmatists slumped forward, blood pouring onto the desk.

That year the death rate in Munich dropped to twenty-two per thousand—the equal, at long last, of London's.

THE FORGOTTEN HERO OF YELLOW FEVER

In the beginning, Jesse W. Lazear was fortunate. He was born with a combination of two of the most important American advantages, money and pedigree. His great-great-grandfather Lazear had immigrated to the New World in 1692 and did well for himself until he was scalped by Virginia Indians in 1730. Grandfather Lazear, for whom Jesse was named, had once represented Green County, Pennsylvania, in the U.S. Congress. Jesse's father was wealthy, and his mother was the former Miss Charlotte S. Clayland Pettigrew, daughter of the mayor of Pittsburgh.

As a young gentleman born in 1886 he was protected from the sweatshops, and he suffered from poor nutrition only when camping. When he went barefoot it was by choice and not necessity. He learned how to ride at an early age, and how to dress for riding. He learned to tell a tablespoon from a soup spoon, and how to use a finger bowl. When he fought with other boys he didn't kick, scratch, bite, or hit below the belt, and he assumed his opponent would follow the same rules of fairness.

His life was not without risk, however. Even wellborn

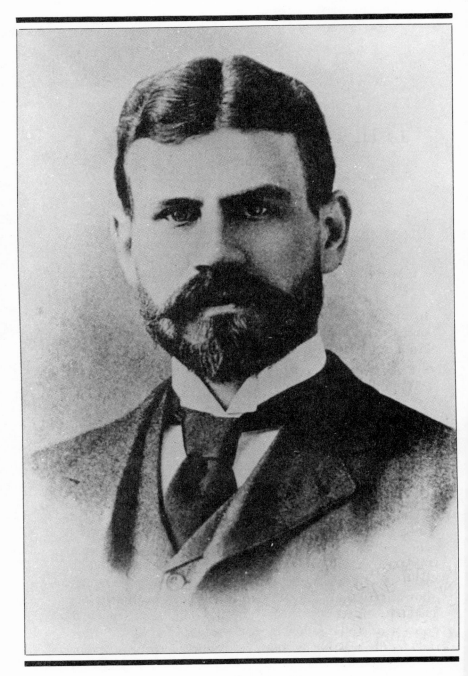

DR. JESSE LAZEAR

babies died of typhoid, diphtheria, cholera, and smallpox, and sometimes yellow fever would bubble out of the Spanish pesthole of Havana and descend on some unfortunate port city like Jesse's home, Baltimore. Then the luckless became feverish, their skin turned yellow, they began to spew up black vomit, and they died. Neither wealth nor family name nor mother's love could protect him from yellow fever, but where those things failed him he had luck.

As a young lad Jesse wasn't told exactly what yellow fever was, of course. But he perceived at an early age that whatever it was, grown-ups were terrified of it. Even his father, who wasn't supposed to be afraid of anything, seemed . . . well . . . subdued at the mention of it. Whatever it was, it came from some faraway place called Havana and it was kept at bay only by God's grace. The family went to church regularly.

In time, little Jesse had a new baby brother, then a second, then a third. All were healthy.

When Jesse was mature enough, he was packed up and sent off to boarding school. This rude eviction from the nest was a shock, as it was to all of his peers, but he survived it. He studied Latin, geometry, history, and science. He learned to sit still and be silent when an adult spoke. He learned mathematics and about Napoleon. He learned about biology and how the dreaded yellow fever rose from the filthy squalor of Havana.

In this context the Spanish seemed somehow . . . evil. The Cubans wanted to evict their oppressors from their country, and many brave young Cuban men had sacrificed their lives in that cause, but so far their efforts had failed. Cuba was in the Caribbean. It was subject to the Monroe Doctrine. Monroe had been the fifth president of the United States. There were nineteen states. The capital of Rhode Island was Providence. The square of the hypotenuse of a right triangle was equal to the sum of the squares of the two adjacent sides.

At least he could spend summers with his grandparents, who lived at a retirement estate in the rolling, forested countryside north of Baltimore, where the July breezes were cool and where the wily brown trout would sometimes take a black and gold fly. There were always plenty of squirrels and an occasional rabbit to hunt. There were horse races and crab feasts and sometimes trips downtown to gawk at the wharves and ships and the sweating black bodies of the stevedores. As he grew older there were also formal parties where he was expected to practice his skills at meeting and wooing the proper members of the opposite sex.

The social system into which Jesse was born didn't necessarily produce gentlemen but, by all accounts, in Jesse's case it did. He understood that he was privileged, and he acknowledged that he owed a debt to his fellowman. He would, he promised himself, fulfill it.

As Teddy Roosevelt would later point out, the era in which Jesse grew from boy to man was one of inexplicable peace. Soldiers were bored and their trade fell somewhat into disrepute. Young men who might have felt called to the military academies went instead into engineering and the peace, when it inevitably ended, would leave a legacy of bridgebuilders.

Jesse Lazear had a fine mind and a solid grasp of mathematics, and he could have been an engineer, but in boarding school he finally got his first glimpse down the barrel of a microscope. He was overwhelmed by the large number of beasties to be found residing in a single drop of pond water. He read about heroes like Robert Koch, who were explaining cholera and the other great diseases, and were laying the foundation for microbiology. For Jesse, biology beckoned, and while he was still too young to

comprehend the details he understood that the new frontier was tropical medicine.

In 1877, for instance, a scientist named Patrick Manson
had discovered something very strange about filariasis. Filariasis, better known as elephantiasis, caused an arm or a
leg (or worse, a sexual organ) to swell to huge proportions.
It was a strange disease to begin with, and now Manson
had shown that it was caused by a microscopic parasite
spread by a mosquito. A bug! Imagine! Imagine such a
fiendishly complex trick of nature! Mosquito to man, man
to mosquito, mosquito to man . . .

Manson's work was widely discussed, but young Jesse
wouldn't have heard of another scientist, one Carlos
Finlay, who was doing similar work involving mosquitoes
and yellow fever. For one thing, Carlos was in Cuba, and
Cuba (as everyone knew) was not exactly a vital center of
scientific progress. Besides, what the man was saying was
obviously preposterous, and he couldn't prove a word of
it. Finlay's work had been published, but it was spoken of
with scorn—and never mentioned around impressionable
students like Jesse.

As the years passed and his classmates flirted with first
one profession and then another, Jesse's ambition remained rock solid. He graduated from high school and
enrolled at Washington and Jefferson College in Pennsylvania, where he joined the snobbish Phi Kappa Psi frater-
nity. In the summer, at his grandfather's estate, he learned
to ride to hounds.

In his third year he switched his enrollment to the recently opened Johns Hopkins University, which was finally offering the aristocrats of Baltimore a means to give
their children a quality education close to home. Though
there had been doubts at first, the new university was
rapidly earning a reputation for excellence and, best of all
from Jesse's point of view, there were indications that the

institution was prepared to invest heavily in medicine and might even open a medical school. It would be a good place, Jesse's father agreed, for a prospective doctor to study.

As the years passed in society balls and fox hunts, friends and family, music and language, history and mathematics, poetry and comparative anatomy, Jesse and his classmates were caught up in the romance of the tropics. Downtown Baltimore smelled of spices and hemp. Steamships brought bananas from Cuba, exotic fruits from Hawaii, and coffee from South America, and the merchant seamen and travelers carried strange tales of adventure and heroism, of cannibal fish in the Amazon, silver in the high Andes, treasure and curses in the jungle-choked ruins of the Maya.

It all had the sense of tropical opportunity, of great works waiting to be performed, of adventure and fortune. The Frenchmen who had built the great Suez Canal through the African desert were being lionized, though there was a rumor . . . Those same engineers were now working to duplicate their feat in Central America and build a canal across the Isthmus of Panama, but the rumor said the workmen there were being drained of strength by malaria and killed by yellow fever. Nobody knew what caused either one, though medical scientists were working almost desperately to find out. The tropics must somehow be made habitable for the white man and his laborers, and doctors who tackled the problem were special heroes.

In 1889, when Lazear received his bachelor's degree, the Johns Hopkins Medical School had begun hiring high-level doctors and scientists, but wasn't yet open to medical students. Jesse's next choice was the Columbia University Medical School in New York. Columbia was a long way from home, on the one hand, but on the other its faculty included several well-known experts on tropical medicine. So that autumn he went to New York to begin the first year of the hazing and drudgery that characterized medical schools of the era.

Though Jesse's training had made him adept in social situations and rewarded him with many acquaintances, he always maintained an inner reserve and his friendships were rare and widely spaced. His reputation as a loner followed him into medical school but there, in the almost battlefield intimacy, he met a young Cuban student, Aristides Agramonte y Simoni, who was almost as reserved as he. Somehow, their defenses canceled out and the two became fast friends. They sat together in lectures, complained to one another about professors, and argued theories of tropical diseases.

To Lazear, Agramonte represented the best of an exotic and brave people. Agramonte was an aristocrat and the son of a great patriot, Eduardo, who had fought the hated Spanish in Cuba's failed revolution. If most of the callow and barbarian medical students didn't know what that meant, Agramonte never forgot it for a moment. He carried himself with dignity, refused to engage in the more childish pranks of medical school, and vowed quietly to return, somehow, to his native land, and to aid his people. Agramonte had the one thing that Jesse had been denied: a heroic dream.

As Jesse memorized the anatomy of the triceps muscle and dissected the ocular nerve out of the head of a dead pauper, he also absorbed an education, via Agramonte, on the subject of the Cuban nation.

He learned for one thing not to judge the Cuban people by their current sad and oppressed state. If yellow fever came from Havana, then consider the filthy condition of the city, caught as it was beneath the heel of the conquistador. If there was poverty in Cuba . . . ask yourself a question: Would the United States be so prosperous, clean, and disease free if its affairs were managed in distant London?

If Lazear felt a bond of friendship with Agramonte, he couldn't help but feel one with Agramonte's people as well. Who could resist admiring a feisty people that wanted to follow in America's footsteps and mount a revolution against its colonial master?

And so Lazear's medical school years passed in a very normal fashion. He shared drudgery and camaraderie, ached with heartbreaking sorrow for the patients who died, repressed a shudder when he met the dog he would have to anesthetize with chloroform and then operate on. As the years passed each student chose, or drifted into, some special interest. Some spent what little free time they had down in obstetrics, assisting in the birth of babies. Others worked in the anatomy suites. Jesse and Agramonte hung around the laboratories, eagerly volunteering to do anything that needed doing in the general proximity of a microscope.

When they graduated, Lazear and Agramonte parted sorrowfully, promising to write often, fearing the promises would prove false, the pain of departure made bearable only by excited anticipation of the future.

Jesse spent the next two years as a junior assistant in medicine at Bellevue Hospital in New York, where he concentrated his studies on the new fields of bacteriology and immunology. Then, to broaden his experience, he

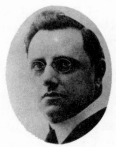

DR. ARISTIDES AGRAMONTE

Courtesy Public Affairs Office, Walter Reed Army Medical Center, Washington, D.C.

spent the winter of 1894–1895 in Europe. His mother, of course, accompanied him.

That winter his life continued its storybook pattern and peaked in a classic Victorian romance. On an excursion to Munich he met a young woman from San Francisco, who was on vacation with her parents. Her name was Mabel Houston and she had large expressive eyes that made Jesse's head go fuzzy, a power shared by her blond hair and great skill at listening attentively whenever Jesse spoke. Jesse, who hadn't had anyone to talk to since he parted with Agramonte, blurted out his feelings to her. In return, she opened up to him. They rode a gondola in Venice, walked in the rain in Florence, toasted their love with wine in Switzerland.

Then Mabel's parents took her back to San Francisco, leaving Jesse to dutifully spend spring in Paris with his mother. Even a storybook life has its flaws.

With the time rapidly approaching when he must choose a discipline and commit himself to it, Jesse's interest settled on malaria. Malaria had its impact in the United States, but it was in the tropics that it stood against the tide of civilization. It felled missionaries in Africa, traders in Brazil, sailors in the South Pacific. In Central America it had teamed up with yellow fever to destroy the French dream of a canal between the Atlantic and the Pacific.

In descriptive terms, a great deal was known about malaria. It never occurred in the winter or at very high altitudes. It was characterized by a fever that came and went with a deadening regularity. In the most common form the fever recurred every three days, and in a variant every four. It was common in marshy areas but it wasn't caused by swamp gas and miasmas, as people like Max von Pettenkofer had thought. In 1880 a French Army surgeon, Charles Laveran, discovered that malaria patients all harbored a tiny parasite in their bloodstreams.

The single-celled parasites were fascinating things to see

under the microscope. You had to know how to stain them, for otherwise they couldn't be seen in their hiding places, inside the red corpuscles. But with a special dye they could be turned blue, which made them stand out clearly against the red background. You had to look for them—they weren't in all the blood cells—but when you found them they were obvious.

They were in the form of a loop, with a thickened segment that had a prominent dot in the middle of it. . . . In Jesse's world, they looked like nothing so much as signet rings. They reproduced themselves inside the bloodstream, not sexually but by division, until the blood cell was nothing but a mass of signet rings. Then it exploded, seeding the rings into the bloodstream to infect other cells.

Looking at the parasites sometimes gave Jesse a strange feeling. To think that such a creature, so apparently simple, was responsible for so much misery! What a thing it would be to help prevent or cure it!

The answers were to be found in the missing pieces of the puzzle. It was clear how the parasite was passed from blood cell to blood cell, but how did it pass from one bloodstream to another? It was clear that the parasite could reproduce by dividing, but shouldn't it have a sexual phase as well? To lack a sexual phase would seem to contradict evolutionary theory. Such a well-adapted species couldn't occur without the constant mixing of genes produced by sexual exchanges. Either evolutionary theory was wrong, or . . . or the rings went somewhere else to mate.

The Johns Hopkins Medical School was a logical place for Lazear to pursue his specialty. The new school, going all out to attract top talent, had snared some bright young stars. There were Osler in medicine, Halsted in surgery, Kelly in gynecology, Flexner in bacteriology, and Welch in pathology. It was Welch's group that was studying malaria. Jesse wrote to the university and received an interested reply. A further exchange of letters and visits resulted in a junior faculty appointment.

Jesse was ecstatic. His slightly senior co-workers would include men like William S. Thayer and William G. Mac-Callum; in a letter to Mabel, Jesse wrote that "there is no such group of men anywhere in the world.

"This is a great privilege, to be able to work with such men," he continued, and then added, "I hope you understand how much I am devoted to this work."

As the academic year opened Jesse found himself in charge of the hospital's new clinical laboratory, making him responsible for actually performing most of the tests that the new era of bacteriology had spawned. Along with his technicians he counted the red blood cells in a frame of magnified blood, calculated the blood count, and diagnosed anemia. He scrutinized bone marrow for the cells that characterized leukemia. He examined urine for the bits and pieces of dead cells that would signify a smoldering infection higher in the urinary tract. And, in Baltimore, it was always wise to keep alert for signs of malaria.

Jesse was eager to apply his knowledge to patients, and whenever possible he offered his services to the clinicians. In that way, during his first winter at the medical school he became involved with a patient of Dr. Thayer's. The patient had an inflammation of the heart that seemed to be seeding infection into the bloodstream itself. Collaborating with Dr. Thayer, he cultured a sample from the patient's bloodstream and identified an alien organism. It was a gonococcus, the venereal disease agent. It turned out that for some reason the disease had gone to the heart lining and, from there, was seeding bacteria into the bloodstream.

Jesse's part in the discovery gave him a wonderful feeling. He wrote to Mabel about it.

Though most of his energy went into his work and into

his developing relationship with a woman a continent
away, Jesse didn't forget Agramonte. The headlines
wouldn't let him.

Another Cuban revolution began the year Jesse had
come to Hopkins. The forces of the revolution were fighting in the mountains. There had been heavy losses to U.S.
investments, and so the newspapers were full of detailed
reports. Editorials pointed out that the United States, if it
was serious about taking over the failed Panama Canal
project from the French, would need Cuba as a base of
operations. The Monroe Doctrine was a topic of discussion. The Spanish were interlopers.

The American public was in sympathy with the aims of
the Cuban people, and none of that sympathy was more
sincere than Jesse Lazear's. At the same time, Cuba was
more distant, in his heart, than San Francisco. He went
west that summer, to visit Mabel's family, and when he
returned in the fall he had a bride on his arm. There was a
round of congratulatory parties and then the new couple
rented an apartment on Lanvale Street. Jesse went back to
work.

In some ways the next year, 1897, was a vintage one for
Jesse. It was the year, for instance, in which the Cuban
revolutionaries won battle after battle against the Spanish,
pushing them into the westernmost provinces. Jesse kept
abreast of developments via the newspapers. At long last,
victory seemed close at hand for Agramonte's people, and
Jesse rejoiced for them.

It was also a year of conquest and excitement in Lazear's
own field of tropical medicine. A British scientist stationed
in India, Dr. Ronald Ross, discovered malaria parasites in
the bellies and salivary glands of a specific type of swamp
mosquito, the *Anopheles*. Was that where the parasites
went to breed? Lazear's fellow Hopkins scientist Mac-
Callum demonstrated that the answer was yes. The signet

rings couldn't spread or reproduce effectively without the *Anopheles* mosquito. If the mosquito could be eliminated, perhaps by draining swamps, malaria could theoretically be prevented.

Jesse absorbed each new fact with excitement. Mosquitoes had been a subject of increasing interest since the discovery that one variety was responsible for the spread of elephantiasis, so the Hopkins library had literature on them. That literature expanded rapidly as the implications of the malaria work caught on.

It was fortunate that mosquitoes were easy to raise. The eggs of the common mosquito could be found floating in the gutters just outside the Hopkins medical school. They could be sucked into an eyedropper and hatched in a bell jar. They could be dissected under a low-power microscope. Suddenly everybody had a mosquito colony, or knew someone who did. Some had even been able to get their hands on the potentially deadly *Anopheles* type.

The mosquito was just the sort of thing that interested young Jesse. It was really a remarkable creature. As an egg, it floated on the water and ate nothing. As a larva, it swam and ate algae. As an adult, it flew and ate fruit.

What made it so important, of course, was the female mosquito's taste for blood. The males didn't bite, but the female's long mouth consisted of six flexible needles, called stylets, encased in a protective sheath.

The process was all very highly evolved. The mosquito's saliva contained an anticoagulant, which, after the stylets had located and pierced a blood vessel, was injected to prevent clotting. Then, certain that clots wouldn't clog her plumbing, she sucked up as many red blood cells as her expandable abdomen could hold. Though she could breed without red cells in her belly, their presence helped ensure more and healthier eggs, and nature had equipped her with an insatiable thirst for blood.

If she was an *Anopheles* mosquito, and if her victim contained the malaria parasites, they entered her belly with the blood cells, mated, and lived for a short while in cysts in her tissues. Then their offspring moved into her salivary glands, from which they entered their next human victim.

It was a life cycle that came with inherent complexities. It was only the female *Anopheles* that was dangerous, and only if she had bitten a malaria victim. Even then she wasn't dangerous until about eight or ten days passed, giving the parasites time to move into the salivary glands. Then and only then did her bite turn deadly.

Everyone working in the field of malaria research felt buoyed by the pace of developments. Even Jesse's own work, which involved finding a better stain for the signet ring parasite, seemed to become more urgent and important.

The year was also one of excitement in related fields of inquiry. Most notably, an Italian scientist named Giuseppe Sanarelli announced that he had isolated bacteria from the bloodstream of a yellow-fever victim. Sanarelli named the new creatures *Bacillus icteroides*, which translates as the "yellow jaundice germ."

In the United States the news was greeted with almost as much jubilation as was the discovery that mosquitoes carried malaria. Yellow fever didn't have the worldwide importance of malaria, but in the Western Hemisphere regions where it was found, it had had a dramatic impact on history. Napoleon had decided to unload the Louisiana territory cheap after yellow fever devastated his armies in the Caribbean. It was yellow fever that had ultimately foiled the French attempt to build a canal across Panama, and it was yellow fever that now threatened American plans to do the same thing. If a yellow-fever bacterium had indeed been found, experiments with it should point the way to a method of prevention.

The surgeon general at the time was George Sternberg, a bacteriologist who had himself devoted much of his research to a fruitless search for a yellow-fever bacterium. He ordered that experiments on *Bacillus icteroides* begin at once.

Sternberg was an admirer of Welch, at the Hopkins, and he chose one of Welch's former students, Walter Reed, to direct the project. The decision sent a wave of excitement through the Hopkins medical school faculty, since everyone in the department either knew Reed personally or knew of him. Suddenly a Hopkins doctor couldn't conduct a casual conversation without some detailed knowledge of yellow fever.

Reed was fifteen years Jesse's senior and had left Baltimore four years before Jesse's return, but it gave the young man a good feeling to see a Hopkins man do important things in the world of microbiology. For one thing, Reed's appointment boded well for Welch's other students, including Jesse himself.

But the claimed yellow-fever bacteria, when they were examined in Reed's laboratory, failed to measure up. Sanarelli's germ, Reed was finally forced to conclude, was nothing more than the "hog cholera" bacillus, an animal disease that occasionally appeared in cultures to embarrass a sloppy scientist. Hog cholera bacteria were very hardy, and if the scientist didn't wash his hands . . . It was the kind of mistake a medical student would make. Privately, there were caustic words for Sanarelli's methods.

While the discovery didn't do anything for the human condition, it did demonstrate that the Hopkins, and Welch's people in particular, and Walter Reed most of all, were public health experts to be reckoned with. Reed was a court favorite and that gave Lazear, who had no reputation at all, a hero to admire and something to aspire to.

When it came to building his own reputation, Jesse needed all the inspiration he could get. On that front, the

year 1897 wasn't such a good one. That was the year that
Dr. Thayer published his paper on the gonococcal infection of the heart, the medical mystery that Jesse had
helped to solve.

The paper was perfectly correct. Jesse agreed with
everything Dr. Thayer said. The only thing that was
missing was Jesse's name. Thayer had given him no credit
at all.

Jesse tried to be philosophical and to remember his
junior standing, and he was encouraged when Thayer did
add his name to a second paper. As the winter of 1897–
1898 passed he supervised the laboratory, worked on finding a better stain for malarial parasites, tried not to think
too much about gonococcal infections of the heart, and
kept close track of the news from Cuba.

The United States seemed about to come down on the
side of the Cuban rebels, whose offensive always seemed
on the verge of success, and the pages of the Baltimore *Sun*
were crammed with news from the Caribbean. When the
Spanish ambassador was reported to have made some dis-
paraging comments about President McKinley, the nation's editorial pages bristled. In April, the *Maine* was
sunk, and it was war.

All across America, men clamored to be accepted for
military service. In May, the intrepid George Dewey defeated the Spanish in the far Philippines. In Cuba, The-
odore Roosevelt led the charge up San Juan Hill. By

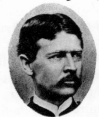

DR. WALTER REED
Courtesy National Library of Medicine

August the Spanish had fled Cuba, and the fighting was all over.

The American victory had been won with a cost of only a few hundred casualties, but as the official reports reached Washington it became clear that there was little cause for celebration. Disease raged in the Army's volunteer training camps. For each American who had died of a Spanish musket ball, several hundred had succumbed to illness.

As the magnitude of the disaster became apparent, apprehension spread through the American high command. The surgeon general summoned his bright young protégé, Walter Reed, and put him in charge of a commission to assess the medical situation. Reed went to work immediately, and within weeks he was back in Washington with exhaustive case studies that traced the spread of disease through the camps.

Most of the deaths were being caused by typhoid, Reed said. He argued that typhoid was caused by the "four Fs"—filth, feces, fingers, and flies—and that the Army camps were being too lax about sanitation.

The eventual result was a crackdown in the enforcement of the Army's sanitary regulations and a satisfying drop in the death rate. Because of his work on typhoid Reed would become a medical hero, the doctor-scientist who could do anything.

As Lazear followed the news, it seemed that everybody who was anybody was involved, somehow, in the Cuban action. Even his old friend Agramonte was there, as part of the effort to clean up Havana.

After the war the United States had resolved to sanitize the Spanish pesthole. The project would demonstrate the benefits of inter-American cooperation, and would have the side effect of putting a lid on yellow fever and thus protecting U.S. ports.

In applying for his appointment to the clean-up team,

Agramonte pointed to the fact that he was a microbiologist with experience in the New York City Health Department, and that his work with urban diseases made him a logical choice.

He was also able to argue that, because he had been raised in Cuba, he was immune to yellow fever. The disease was so common on the island that Cuban children either died of it or survived it, and never contracted it again. The epidemics among adults, he reminded the commission, were always confined to the immigrant populations.

Now Agramonte was in Havana, in uniform, a "contract surgeon" in charge of a microbiology laboratory, making himself count in the world, Walter Reed was in the thick of the typhoid cleanup, and Jesse Lazear . . .

Jesse Lazear was home, safe, in Baltimore, peering at signet rings through a microscope, making out work schedules for laboratory technicians, learning how to change diapers, thirty-one years old, getting a little flabby, sitting in his office, reading the journal article that described his work with malarial stains.

It was his work, all right. He recognized it as his own. But the name at the top of the page wasn't Jesse Lazear, it was Dr. T. B. Futcher, Jesse's boss. Jesse wasn't even listed as a co-author.

Depressed and disheartened, he wondered about this business of being a contract surgeon for the Army. Did they need any more microbiologists in Cuba?

Yes, he discovered. Yes, they did.

It was February 10, 1900, when the ship carrying Jesse, Mabel, and the baby arrived in Havana. The harbor was full of ships. The docks were alive with sweating, half-naked stevedores. It was a warm, balmy day, with a northeastern breeze, a happy contrast to the Baltimore winter the new Army family had so recently put behind them. Agramonte was waiting for them and the reunion was joyous.

Later the Lazear family traveled by coach the eight miles to Columbia barracks, where they were billeted in a small, square house.

Mabel explored the house with mixed emotions. It was of board-and-batten construction, a style used, in Maryland, only to build barns. She could tell the place had once been painted, but now its decor was best described as . . . weathered. There were no cooking facilities; they would have to eat at the officers' mess. There was also no indoor plumbing. Attempting to be philosophical about the situation, she acknowledged the accommodations were at least superior to the long tents that they had passed on the way in, which housed the Army's enlisted contingent.

While Jesse was at the hospital, checking into his new job, Mabel investigated her surroundings. The creatures in the outhouse seemed a little . . . overwhelming. The other wives advised her that it would be worse when the rainy season came in April or May, and they instructed her on the care and use of mosquito netting. Mabel, who was beginning to swell with her second pregnancy, listened to their tales and reminded herself that she was a good sport.

As February and March passed, the family settled into the routine of the tropics. The exotic fruits almost made up for the insects in the outhouse, and the days were uniformly perfect. At the hospital, a cluster of low buildings made with the same board-and-batten construction as the house, Jesse found conditions tolerable if not good. The hospital was at least kept sparkling clean, and the laboratory was well equipped, considering its remote location.

Jesse spent his days peering through a microscope, looking for malarial parasites and examining the blood of suspected typhoid victims. Typhoid was still a problem, though it was nothing like it had been before Reed's work. If only the Army would learn the value of cleanliness!

The work was varied enough to be interesting. Thanks to the availability of fiery Cuban rum at cheap prices, there were always fights and accidents, and Jesse was frequently called upon to examine the pus from wounds. Gonorrhea was always a problem in the Army and, in the tropics, every week would bring a case of some obscure, exotic disease. Since the rainy season hadn't begun yet, there weren't many fungal infections . . .

Jesse, like all newcomers who arrived during the dry season, was somewhat skeptical of rainy-season tales. After all, Havana didn't get that much more precipitation, on the average, than Baltimore. And what could be so bad about a little rain?

After work, it was good to be able to spend time, once again, with Agramonte. At every opportunity the two sat for hours, discussing world affairs, Cuba, wives, children, senior officers—and tropical medicine.

As anyone could see, conditions in Havana were improving day by day. Typhoid became less of a problem each week, as did malaria. Dr. William Gorgas, who had been appointed to head the clean-up commission, was clearly doing an admirable job and there was an assumption that, as a result, the rainy season this year would bring few cases of yellow fever. Havana would be a far healthier place in the future, without a doubt. That was why Army officers like Jesse had felt safe bringing their wives and children to the island.

But in the old days, Agramonte said, yellow fever had arrived shortly after the first rains. In those times, Cuban parents had special reason to worry about a child that hadn't yet survived its first rainy season. The big epidemics, though, raged among the Spanish immigrants, who died wholesale from it . . . presumably because of their atrocious sanitation.

It was difficult for the newcomers to believe the stories. It probably hadn't been quite as bad as all that and, besides, with American medicine on the scene and the defiling Spaniards driven out, yellow fever was no longer a worry . . . unless, of course, the mosquito man was correct.

The mosquito man was Carlos Finlay, the Havana doctor, who thought yellow fever was caused by mosquitoes.

It was really too bad about Finlay. Agramonte said he had been a bright light of Cuban medicine; he could have been a Cuban intellectual hero . . . but because of his obsession with mosquitoes Finlay was instead a laughingstock.

March ended and April began. The promised rains came, hammering down on the tin roofs, and the air turned thick and steamy. Huge spiders hid under the woodwork, while clouds of mosquitoes appeared from nowhere and hovered around the houses. Mabel suddenly found herself totally absorbed in mastering the skills of using and maintaining mosquito netting.

There seemed to be an infinite variety of mosquitoes, big ones and little ones, loud ones and silent ones, fat ones and thin ones, and while none of them were friendly the worst were tiny things, malevolently intelligent creatures that were capable of finding the smallest tear in the netting. They seemed to live in the house itself and they bit without pain. It was only after they flew off that the bite hurt like the stab of the knife. There were strange birdcalls from the brush and frightening shapes scurried, half seen, across the porch. The baby cried in the oppressive heat and Mabel's pregnancy made her more sensitive to discomfort. She developed an edge in her voice.

At the hospital, Jesse heard that there was a case of

yellow fever among the Spanish immigrants, who, now that the war was over, had resumed their flow into Havana. The following week there were several cases. Then a soldier got sick and, somewhat later, another.

As Jesse tried to comprehend the surprising news, the flaw in everyone's assumptions about yellow fever became painfully obvious. The link between filth and yellow fever had never been more than a guess, and though it seemed logical at the time it seemed less so now. What if the cause was something else? What if Cuba, which was now home to thousands of nonimmune American soldiers and their families, experienced another epidemic?

Jesse tried not to sound as alarmed as he really was. It would be far better, he told Mabel, for her to have the baby in a proper hospital back in the United States. In October Jesse could take leave and come home to get her.

Mabel, who probably would have rejected the idea outright before the start of the rainy season, was now easy to convince. Within the week Jesse stood on a dock in Havana, watching a steamer carry his wife and child out of the harbor. October seemed a long time away.

Events soon proved Jesse's prudence wise. After a few sporadic cases, yellow fever struck the immigrant population with a terrible force. Suddenly the Americans realized that the stories hadn't been exaggerated by the natives after all. By June the harbor was empty of ships and the sinister "yellow jack" quarantine flag flapped wetly from the harbor master's staff. The rain, by now, was almost constant.

Life at the hospital was hectic, and Jesse had little time to sulk over his loneliness. As the rains continued the fever-wracked soldiers arrived at the hospital in a constant stream. Some walked in, but many arrived in horse-drawn ambulances.

They were brought to a hastily established admitting

area, and the first task was to clean them up—the bathing facilities at the camp were almost nonexistent and most of the patients stank. Laboring under the direction of frantic nurses, orderlies filled metal bathtubs with water. Hot water was a problem until one of the medical officers found some pipe, served a "midnight requisition" for it, and set up a makeshift solar heater.

Jesse, in the meantime, was using his laboratory skills to help sort the patients according to disease. The problem was that a lot of tropical diseases besides yellow fever began with a bout of fever, and most of them were more common during the rainy season. Malaria was one, and so was typhoid. The rains also brought an epidemic of an intestinal disease called dengue fever, a nonfatal illness that, at its onset, could easily be confused with yellow fever.

Jesse and his fellow physicians diagnosed the soldiers mostly by a process of elimination. If the victim had malaria, Jesse could find the signet ring parasites in his blood. If typhoid was the problem, the pathologists would get a positive result from cultures. If it wasn't malaria, and it wasn't typhoid, and it wasn't dengue, well . . . that was too bad.

Yellow fever had a macabre way of toying with its victim before killing him. For three days there was fever and chills, followed by a marked improvement. The temperature fell and the soldier could sit up and talk to the nurses. He could think, if it pleased him to fantasize, that the worst was past. Maybe, he could tell himself, it had been influenza. Or perhaps a light touch of malaria. Or some unnamed tropical thing, of which there were many.

But on the fourth day yellow fever returned with a vengeance. Beads of sweat popped out on the victim's skin as the fever returned and climbed steadily to 103, 104, 105 . . . and then the chills came and the victim's teeth chattered and he begged for covers . . . only to kick them away again when the fever returned.

Outside, the rains came down. Screen doors slammed as the orderlies carried out the bodies and brought in new patients. Mosquitoes buzzed. Glazed eyes stared at the tent fabric, seeing nothing.

Slowly, the patient's skin turned yellow and patches of the inside of his mouth began to ooze blood. Nausea came, and passed, and returned. There was a pan by each victim's bed to catch the black vomit, a mixture of blood and digestive juices.

Perhaps two thirds of the patients eventually recovered, though their survival had little if anything to do with the ministrations of the physicians. Those who lived did so, perhaps, because they had strong immune systems. Or maybe they had gotten a weaker dose of . . . of . . . of whatever it was. Or perhaps, as far as Jesse knew, they recovered because God willed it.

For those who didn't live, the jaundiced skin became yellower and yellower. Jesse knew the end was near when his tests detected that protein had begun to leak out of the blood, through the kidney membranes, and into the urine. Shortly after that, the kidneys shut down and the flow of urine ceased.

When the kidneys died, so did hope. The wracking hiccups began. If the patient was lucky, he started picking at the bedclothes and went into a coma at about that time. If he was not so fortunate, consciousness faded into delirium and he screamed and cried out in his living nightmare until just before death, which usually occurred between the sixth and the ninth day.

And so for the doctors one day of labor blended into another, and the post's graveyard expanded. The rains came daily, in the afternoon, and when they were over steam rose from the hot ground. In the evenings there were clouds of mosquitoes and some of them even got into the hospital, despite the screening on the doors and windows. Overcoming his exhaustion, Jesse wrote often to Mabel. May ended. June began.

In Washington the surgeon general, alarmed over the yellow-fever epidemic, had decided to find the elusive yellow-fever bacteria once and for all. Walter Reed, who had become known as Surgeon General Sternberg's wonder boy as a result of his typhoid work, had been named to head a four-man yellow-fever commission in Havana.

Reed would, of course, bring James Carroll. Carroll was a bacteriologist who, over the years, had become Reed's right-hand man. Once Reed and Carroll reached Havana, they would need two more commission members, doctors who knew the local conditions and who could be relied on in a laboratory. Agramonte was an obvious choice, especially since he was immune. And then there was that young, super-serious fellow, Jesse Lazear . . . Reed, Carroll, Agramonte, and Lazear. That would serve well, for a beginning.

Shortly after the decision was made in Washington, Jesse was at his microscope, as he often was, when he sensed someone standing over him. He looked up. It was the hospital's commanding officer and he had a dispatch in his hand.

Lazear read the message again and again, his heart racing. The more he thought about it, the more he became convinced that this was his long-awaited opportunity to make his mark as a scientist.

The days passed slowly for Jesse and Agramonte as they awaited the arrival of Reed and Carroll, and when the ship reached Havana they were waiting on the dock to greet their new boss.

When Reed was in Washington he often traveled to Baltimore to consult with Welch, so Jesse had seen him from afar. He had always seemed like a dignified man, but as his reputation had grown so had the aura of competence and authority that surrounded him. Even had he been wearing civilian clothes, which he certainly was not, his walk would have identified him instantly as a military officer. Carroll did Reed's bidding, opening doors for him, taking notes, and obeying him like an enlisted man. It was impossible for Lazear and Agramonte not to take their cue from that.

During their ride to Columbia Barracks, the three junior men maintained a respectful silence as Reed scrutinized the wet countryside. At the barracks there was a welcoming committee, and Reed was occupied for several hours making small talk with various officers and then getting settled in his room. Finally, the four commission members were alone on the veranda.

Reed did most of the talking, and sometimes he seemed to be directing the conversation inward, thinking aloud, summarizing for himself as well as for Carroll, Agramonte, and Lazear.

In the sense that the Spanish-American War had been an opportunity for combat officers, the yellow-fever epi-

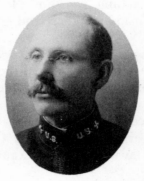

DR. JAMES CARROLL

Courtesy National Library of Medicine

demic was a godsend for the medical corps. What made it even more perfect was that Surgeon General Sternberg had a special interest in tracking down the yellow-fever bacteria—a fact that would become very significant once success had been achieved. Reed obviously relished the challenge to come and had great confidence about its probable outcome. In the meantime, the commission might as well settle in and make itself comfortable—this investigation was likely to last a year or two.

Jesse stood quietly, listening. Despite the failure of the Havana cleanup to prevent the outbreak of yellow fever, then, there was still an unspoken assumption that the disease was spread in some fashion similar to typhoid. It was presumed to be a bacterial infection passed somehow by filth. Reed didn't say "filth," of course. "Fomites" was the proper medical word. Feces. Vomit. Sweat. Urine. They produced a sort of a . . . call it a miasma.

In the conversation, the miasmology of Pettenkofer and the microbiology of Koch and Pasteur formed an uneasy alliance of old and new. Where was the agent of disease important, and how was it influenced by environmental factors? In the end, no one knew.

By the time the meeting drew to a close, Jesse understood that his specific role would be the most minor of the four. Agramonte would study the victims' bodies, do the autopsies, and select bits of tissue for study. Carroll would culture that tissue and try to identify the responsible microbe. Jesse was needed mainly to distinguish the yellow-fever patients from those with malaria, and to help with laboratory work.

After the meeting, there were more officers waiting to be ushered into Reed's presence. Reed talked politely with each one, swapping yellow-fever stories and speculating on the nature of the disease. Jesse sat and listened. The next day, work began.

As the June rains faded into the July rains, Jesse worked diligently in his support role, making certain the other three weren't misled into experimenting on malarial patients. Nothing came of Carroll's initial cultures, but Reed hadn't expected instant success. Perhaps they should try different techniques, or use another stain. Perhaps the bacteria infected the body in some unexpected organ and they hadn't yet cultured the right tissue. Reed had patience and it behooved his juniors to cultivate that attribute as well.

Jesse understood the advantages of plodding, methodical, patient science . . . but he was uneasy nevertheless. The fomite theory seemed, somehow, too pat. He did his work, kept his laboratory notebook carefully, assisted the others in every way he could, and made no complaints. But after hours, his thoughts were his own.

As he considered it, the fomite theory grew weaker and weaker. For one thing, there was Nathaniel Potter. To help quell a panic during a yellow-fever epidemic in the late 1700s, he had argued that the disease wasn't contagious at all. He was so certain of his assertion that he soaked towels in black vomit and the perspiration of yellow-fever patients, wrapped them around his head, and slept with them there. He didn't get yellow fever. A few years later Stubbins Ffirth, at the University of Pennsylvania, had inoculated himself with black vomit and blood from yellow-fever patients, and nothing happened to him, either.

Of course, Jesse had to admit, both men had been doctors, and since they had treated yellow-fever patients they might well have been immune. So it was an open question, but still . . .

There was another thing, too, that nagged at him. One of the visitors after that first meeting with Reed had been Henry Rose Carter, a U.S. Public Health Service officer assigned to the quarantine service. He told Reed he had noticed that yellow-fever epidemics seemed to begin in a rather peculiar way, in a fashion unlike other diseases. First there was one isolated case. Then, three weeks later, there was a cluster of new cases. Subsequent cases appeared constantly, but that first case, for some reason, was separated from the others by a twenty-one-day lag time.

Jesse was intrigued by that but he could tell that Reed, though he had listened politely, was not. When Carter was ready to go, Jesse followed him out the door and engaged him in discussion.

Everything Jesse learned about yellow fever made him suspect that Reed and the rest were in error when they thought in terms of a typhoidlike disease. To Jesse's mind it bore more resemblance to malaria. Malaria even had a lag time—it took a number of days for the parasites to mate in the mosquito and for their offspring to find their way to the salivary gland, and then to the human. In the meantime, the mosquito wasn't infectious.

Perhaps yellow fever, like malaria, had to be spread by a "vector," or agent of some kind. If that was the case you could wrap your head in fomites and never get yellow fever.

Jesse, as his musings and readings progressed, began taking careful notes. It was prudent, he reasoned, to keep those notes in a separate, private notebook. For one thing, while he was pursuing his separate theories on his own time, he certainly didn't want Reed to get the impression that it was interfering with the bacteria-hunting work. Besides, if he struck anything big . . . Jesse tried not to spend much time thinking about it, but this time . . . this time he wanted to get credit for it. He chose a small brown notebook that was easy to carry in his pocket.

As Jesse was puzzling over the problem and collecting his thoughts in his notebook, a pair of yellow-fever experts from Liverpool happened to pass through Havana on their way to Brazil. Their visit was an occasion for all the yellow-fever scientists in Havana to get together for a dinner. For the first time, Jesse met Carlos Finlay.

Carlos Finlay didn't strike Jesse Lazear as the fool he was reputed to be. Though approaching seventy, Finlay still maintained a private practice and carried on research. He was polite, even warm, as he told the others that yellow fever was carried by mosquitoes. He said it as if it were an objective, proven fact.

And it wasn't just any mosquito, Finlay continued. It was one species in particular, a member of the *Stegomyia* group. It was a tiny thing with a peculiar tapered abdomen, and it was the only kind that actually bred in houses. Swamp mosquitoes like those that carried malaria might fly into the house and bite people, but the yellow-fever mosquito lived and bred inside, in the drinking water.

Finlay talked on, absorbed in his own subject. The British scientists seemed to be impressed with the argument— impressed enough, they said, to send a note to the *British Medical Journal.*

The house mosquitoes that Finlay spoke of were fascinating to Jesse. Before evolving to live in humans' houses they had laid their eggs in shallow pools that dried up between rains. They had developed the useful habit of depositing the eggs just above the waterline, so that if the water went down they remained dormant. When the next rainy season began and the pools filled up and the eggs became wet, they hatched into wrigglers, the wrigglers metamorphosed into pupae, and the pupae turned into mosquitoes.

This instinct to lay the eggs above the waterline made it possible for them to thrive in human dwellings. Humans kept a jug of drinking water around the house. The water level got lower, and lower, and lower . . . and then someone refilled it. It was perfect.

Finlay had once had the opportunity, under the Spanish government, to experiment with soldiers. He had found patients with clear cases of yellow fever, let mosquitoes feed on their blood, and then let the mosquitoes bite volunteer soldiers.

The results were consistent with the hypothesis, in that some of the volunteers did become ill. But, Finlay sadly admitted, the results hadn't been very convincing because it didn't seem to be classic yellow fever—none of the soldiers had died. And, since yellow fever was deadly one time in three, Finlay's peers judged that the illnesses, whatever they were, weren't yellow fever.

The medical community hadn't laughed Finlay out of town . . . they didn't do that in the land of machismo. They didn't insult you to your face. They looked embarrassed for him and changed the subject. But Finlay had gotten the message. The irony was that if one of the soldiers had died, it would all have been different.

Someone asked about the most efficient way to raise mosquitoes, about Finlay's theories on lag time, and about his opinion on bacteria. Finlay agreed in principle that there had to be bacteria, all right—or something. He had looked for it, he said, even thought he found it once, but . . . the only thing he was certain of was that yellow fever,

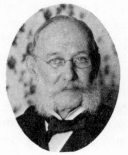

DR. CARLOS FINLAY

Courtesy National Library of Medicine

whatever it was, was transmitted by mosquitoes. He couldn't prove it, but in his mind that was the only thing that made sense.

Jesse rode back to the hospital, lost in thought. Reed hadn't seemed particularly interested in Finlay's theories at dinner, but the two had talked briefly afterward and arranged for Reed's commission to visit Finlay at home for further discussions.

Jesse suspected that Reed was simply trying to cover all bases and to do a courtesy to the old scientist, but Jesse was finding the mosquito theory more and more enticing. After all, the microbe hunters hadn't found anything revealing in their cultures—so the mosquitoes were worth trying, if for no other reason than that nothing else seemed to work.

When the appointed day came, Finlay welcomed the Americans into his expansive house and offered them wine. Reed listened, with a pleasant and interested expression on his face, while the old man discussed his mosquito theory in depth. Finlay, though persistent, didn't become argumentative.

It was all very interesting, Reed said.

Perhaps.

Who knows?

And certainly, if Dr. Lazear was willing to take care of them, the mosquitoes should cause no disruption. Afterward Reed accepted a gift of mosquito eggs.

The group said its good-byes and headed back for the Columbia Barracks. By common consent, Reed, Carroll, and Agramonte immediately changed the subject to other matters, to culture preparation and the nature of bacteria. But Lazear had a small envelope of mosquito eggs in his pocket and could think of nothing else. Back at the barracks he went immediately to his laboratory.

Immersed in water, the eggs turned into tiny wrigglers that hung beneath the water's surface, breathing through tubes. These presently turned into pupae that darted through the water until finally bursting. One by one the mosquitoes emerged, perching precariously on rafts formed by the pupae shells, their wet wings catching the light and splitting it into rainbows. Then, when dry, they flew upward and lit on the glass wall of the test tube.

Even with the naked eye Jesse could distinguish the elaborate antennae of the male, designed to home in on the hum of the female's wings, from the simpler antennae of the female. He fed them on bits of fruit. That satisfied their nutritional requirements, but only whetted the female's lust for blood.

So that the mosquitoes could complete their life cycle in the most realistic way possible, Lazear fed the females by the simple expedient of uncorking the test tubes and holding them against his arm. The female mosquitoes inside sensed his body warmth and, flying expertly through the atmospheric heat eddies above the skin, landed.

Jesse watched thoughtfully as a mosquito folded back the sheath that protected her slender mouthparts—six sharp but flexible hypodermic needles, the stylets. Each stylet was pierced by two channels, one for injecting saliva and the other for sucking.

The saliva had acquired a second characteristic in the Cuban house mosquito. The human is better equipped than most animals to swat a mosquito, and so the survivors developed a saliva protein that served to deaden the victim's nerve endings.

As Jesse watched, the mosquito's stylets felt expertly for his nerve, found them, injected the painkiller, and then proceeded to pierce a capillary and suck his blood. As the seconds passed, her abdomen filled. Only after she had departed did Jesse begin to feel the sting and itch, as the painkiller wore off and his immune system reacted to the saliva.

The agents of at least two diseases, elephantiasis and

malaria, could travel in mosquito saliva. Could yellow
fever be a third?

It wasn't difficult to get the commission to agree that
human volunteers could be used. For one thing, everyone
who hadn't had yellow fever would eventually get it, and
when you did, your chances of survival were probably
better if you got immediate medical attention. The volunteers, since they would be watched constantly, would naturally get that. Any possible criticism of the project was
defused when Reed, Carroll, and Lazear agreed to be
among the volunteers. Agramonte, of course, was already
immune.

The day after the commission approved the use of volunteers, however, Reed was called back to Washington for
discussions with the surgeon general and the experiments
had to proceed without him.

The experimental design was simple. Lazear took test
tubes with hungry females in them to the yellow-fever
wards, chose the sickest patients, and held the mouths of
the tubes against the victims' skin. The mosquitoes, obeying their programmed imperatives, immediately settled
and gorged themselves with blood. Jesse made careful
notes in his brown notebook, recording which mosquito
bit which patient and precisely when.

There had to be a dormancy period, Jesse reasoned,
which would explain the observation that the first case in
an epidemic wasn't followed by secondary cases for some
time. He waited for a week to pass, and then another, and
then he let the mosquitoes begin to gorge on the blood of
the volunteers. Jesse had planned to use nine subjects—
seven soldiers, himself, and Carroll—but he had to settle
for eight because Carroll was nowhere to be found.

The days passed, Jesse keeping careful, detailed notes in
his little brown book. The volunteers lounged in the hospital, flirting with the nurses and leading what, for a soldier, was the good life. He himself felt fine. He teased

Carroll for his absence on mosquito-biting day and Carroll, embarrassed, provided a valid explanation. Next time, he promised.

But on August 25, when Jesse's mosquitoes were ready to bite another group of volunteers, Carroll again turned up missing. Again Jesse went ahead without him, but promised himself to involve Carroll as soon as possible. It looked better, much better, if all the doctors participated.

Jesse counted the days, waiting for one of his second group of volunteers to get sick. None of them did.

Puzzled, brown notebook open, Jesse sat before his mosquito cages and thought through the experiments. He was obviously doing something wrong. But what?

Jesse hadn't wanted his results to be confused by patients who turned out to have malaria and dengue fever, so he had been using only the sickest, late-stage patients. That made sense, too, insofar as those patients were the sickest.

But what if, for some strange and unguessed reason, the yellow-fever agent could be passed only during the first few days of the illness? That would explain why the mosquitoes weren't working.

He could test the idea by feeding mosquitoes on patients who had developed fevers, and then watching each patient while his blood incubated in the mosquito's belly. That would require a lot of record keeping, because he would have to disqualify some mosquitoes when the people they had bitten came down with malaria, dengue, or even typhoid. On the other hand, he could take one mosquito and let her bite several patients who might be in the early stages of yellow fever. That would be simpler, and would require fewer mosquitoes and fewer patients.

A letter arrived from home, informing him that he was the father of a healthy baby boy. It was a cause for fat Cuban cigars all around.

Jesse let a new batch of mosquitoes bite feverish but

undiagnosed patients. By August the twenty-seventh, the
mosquitoes were ready and that same day, at lunch,
Lazear spied Carroll. He sat down beside him, made some
small talk, and then started teasing him.

Lazear told Carroll that he had some very hungry mosquitoes. Poor things . . . one of them hadn't had any
blood for weeks. The desperate insect was terribly hungry, he said. It was a very sad case.

Carroll took another mouthful of food.

It was, Jesse continued throughout the meal, truly sad.
Consider the poor, starving creature, held captive in a test
tube, with nothing to eat but a sliver of banana. . . .

All right, sighed Carroll, as he finished his food and slid
his chair back. Okay. You win.

The two put on their raincoats and walked back to
Jesse's laboratory, chatting about Carroll's cultures of
yellow-fever tissue. There were no results yet, Carroll
said. Nothing. It was very strange, very strange indeed—
there had to be *something* in the autopsy tissue. After all,
yellow fever had killed the donors, hadn't it? And yet,
under the microscope, there was nothing abnormal to be
seen. It didn't make sense.

At the laboratory, Jesse selected a mosquito. Carroll,
still talking about his cultures, stuck out his arm. Jesse
removed the stopper from the test tube and upended it
over the skin. Carroll stopped talking as he watched the
mosquito light and bury its snout in his flesh. Slowly, the
mosquito's abdomen expanded with blood.

When it was done, Carroll rubbed his arm, waved goodbye to Lazear and returned to the commission's more important work, which was the cultures. A few minutes later
Lazear was back at his problem, bent over his own notebook, trying to figure out why the yellow-fever germ was
so elusive. Perhaps, he thought, it needed some special
condition in which to grow, or a special food. . . .

The day passed, and another. Then, on August 29,

while making rounds with the other doctors at the hospital, Carroll felt inexplicably weak. He fell back from the group, forced himself to catch up, fell back again. Finally he excused himself and went out on the porch, where it was a little cooler, to wait for rounds to finish.

After resting he felt better. Malaria? He knew the signs well, and he was unusually tired the following day as well. Malaria? No. Overwork. He told no one.

Jesse, in the meantime, had decided to let the same mosquito that had bitten Carroll feed on another experimental subject as well. On the morning of August 31 he summoned a volunteer soldier, William Dean, and let the mosquito bite him.

On that same day Carroll rose at reveille, sat on the edge of his bed, cradled his head in his hands, and admitted to himself that he wasn't just tired from overwork; he was sick. There was no longer any denying it.

He forced himself to get out of bed, put on his uniform, and slowly made his way to his laboratory. There he took a sample of his own blood, stained it for malarial parasites, and peered at it through the lenses. No signet rings. Nothing. That was a relief.

Perhaps, whatever it was, it would go away.

Throughout the morning Carroll tried to work, but by afternoon the fatigue was overwhelming and a fever had begun. He made an excuse, returned to his room, and went to bed. By evening his fever had risen to 102 and the illness could no longer be concealed. When the fever broke, then returned again on September 2 and climbed to 104, the diagnosis was certain. It was yellow fever.

For Lazear, everything fell into place. Nobody had ever experimented much with early-stage patients, because they couldn't be reliably diagnosed as having yellow fever . . . and yet, Lazear now thought, the early stage was obviously the key.

The joy of the realization was tempered by guilt. Time

and time again, Jesse remembered the scene in the officers' mess, when he had goaded Carroll into letting himself be bitten. Now Carroll was getting sicker by the hour. What if he should die? Lazear kept telling Agramonte that he hadn't done it on purpose, and that he had participated in an earlier experiment himself.

Yet the facts rang hollow. Jesse hadn't gotten sick, but Carroll had; that was all that counted, and as the days passed Carroll got worse and worse.

Yet as a scientist Lazear could do nothing now except use the knowledge, gained at Carroll's expense, wisely. Knowing there would have to be other experiments, Lazear set about infecting more mosquitoes with blood from early-stage patients.

By September 3 Carroll's fever-burned skin had begun to take on the sickening hues of yellow jaundice. The fever rose, and rose some more, and his teeth chattered with the chills. Sometimes he recognized his co-workers and sometimes he didn't. The inside of his mouth bled and he retched black vomit into the waiting pan. Then, on September 7, the fever broke.

Jesse's relief was tempered by a new source of guilt, for Dean, the soldier who had been bitten in the second experiment with Carroll's mosquito, was now sick.

First Carroll, now Dean! Two out of two!

Lazear's experiments, for all practical purposes, had been conducted in secret—or more accurately in obscurity, which had the same effect. Not even Agramonte knew, or seemed to care, what was in the little brown notebook. Though Lazear had talked freely, everyone seemed to think that Carroll's illness, and then Dean's, had been happenstance.

"I rather think I am on the track of the real germ," Lazear wrote to his wife in one of his frequent letters. "But nothing must be said as yet, not even a hint. I have not mentioned it to a soul."

When it became clear that Dean had a mild case of yellow fever and wouldn't die, Jesse was beside himself with relief combined with impatience. But his current crop of mosquitoes hadn't bitten yellow-fever patients until the first week in September, and it would be at least the thirteenth before they would become infectious. Carroll's close brush with death had made Jesse much more conservative; he had decided to do the next series of experiments with guinea pigs, not people, and he was eager to get on with it.

In the meantime, life continued. The rains came down and the soldiers filed into the admitting area of the hospital, feverish and weak, and were bathed and parceled out into the various isolation units. On the eleventh, Carroll weakly got to his feet for the first time. He walked a few steps and then had to lie back down, but it was a healthy sign. Dean's fever broke.

On the thirteenth, the mosquitoes were ready.

Jesse cuddled a guinea pig in the crook of his arm, parted its fur, and pressed the open test tube against its skin. Then he recorked the test tube, returned the animal to its cage, and recorded the inoculation in the brown notebook. Then he did the same with another guinea pig, and another, and another.

The problem was that Jesse had no way of knowing whether guinea pigs were even capable of getting yellow fever. Perhaps it was a strictly human disease, like, say, malaria. Much of Jesse's studies had been on bird malaria, because it was easier to work with. Humans couldn't get bird malaria and birds couldn't get human malaria. What if yellow fever was like that?

It would be far better to use people, but now that Carroll had so dramatically demonstrated the dangers of the experiments, how could Lazear, in all good conscience, ask for volunteers?

Jesse reached for a test tube, checked its label, and made

an entry in the brown notebook. He noted that mosquito had bitten four feverish patients who later turned out to have serious cases of yellow fever. He added some technical details, thought for a moment, wrote some more.

He looked up at the mosquito, thinking. Then he picked up the vial, uncapped it, and held its open end against his skin.

When he wrote to Mabel, he told her only about the guinea pigs. There was no point in worrying her with the other.

The days passed in routine work. Jesse examined slides, did routine research, let more mosquitoes bite more guinea pigs. As the week passed he examined the experimental animals every day, but they seemed healthy. Each day, he sat down and reviewed the latest entries in his notebook.

On September 18, he was rewarded. And the new case wasn't in a guinea pig.

Unlike Carroll, Lazear didn't deny the symptoms. In fact, he welcomed them.

That made his score, with humans at least, three out of three. The results, to his mind, were conclusive. Yellow fever was passed by mosquitoes, but could only be spread by insects that had bitten a patient in the first three days of his illness. Later-stage patients weren't infectious.

As the fever built and began to be punctuated by the icy chills, Jesse reveled in the knowledge. He had solved the problem of yellow fever! He and he alone! There would be no other name on the paper, just J. Lazear! And it would be read, and studied, by everybody in tropical medicine!

He wouldn't tell them yet, though. Not now. He wouldn't make Finlay's mistake.

When Jesse laid out his evidence there would be no argument because there would be no doubt. It would be well thought out, perfectly demonstrated, lucid. But it was difficult to be lucid now. The joy. The fever . . .

Mabel . . . It would be better, perhaps, if Mabel didn't ever understand exactly. . . .

They made him lie down on a stretcher. That was silly. Yellow-fever patients seldom needed a stretcher until the second stage of the disease. He tried to protest but, somehow, couldn't. The world looked different through the fever.

The notebook was in the pocket of his blouse. Good. That was a good place for it; it would be all right there. He couldn't take notes now anyway.

But they were asking him questions.

There was somebody there with gold major's leaves on his collar, major's leaves and a medical corps insignia. Was that William Gorgas? What was Gorgas doing here?

On the third day the temporary respite came, and Jesse's head cleared enough to worry about what he had said while delirious. Had he blurted out anything about mosquitoes? About mosquitoes and yellow fever? He wasn't ready to talk about that yet, but they were asking him questions.

In the momentary clarity, he thought quickly. A half-truth would do.

He told them that yes, he thought yellow fever was transmitted by mosquitoes. And he had been working in the hospital . . . he remembered it clearly . . . and a mosquito had bitten him.

That was it! A mosquito had bitten him accidentally!

He hadn't felt it, of course, but he had seen it, and he hadn't slapped it because he thought it was the wrong kind. Well, the joke was on him. It had been the right kind after all.

Carroll swallowed the story without question, and so did Gorgas. Agramonte looked suspicious but didn't push the issue. The worry, on their end, seemed to be not the experiments but Jesse.

The three, Gorgas, Carroll, and Agramonte, talked

about it in the hallway. Gorgas said it was without a doubt the worst case he had ever seen.

The respite ended and the fever returned. The rain outside sounded like the babbling of the Jones Falls back in Maryland, on his grandfather's farm, where it was autumn. It would soon be the season for quail, and then deer. The geese would fly overhead in big V formations, heading south for faraway exotic places, like Cuba. And then it was winter and there was bone-shaking cold, followed by fever, followed by a season of nausea.

By holding his hands in front of his face Jesse could see that his skin had grown peculiar and yellow, like an Oriental's. Dimly, he realized that the blood in the pan had been vomited up from his own stomach, but the fact was far away.

He would be famous.

In October he would see Mabel and they would celebrate.

October.

October and home were less than a month away; they couldn't tie him here, could they, with gauze around his wrists and ankles? He thrashed and screamed, and there was a cold cloth on his forehead but he didn't notice.

Each day, at the desperate insistence of Carroll and Agramonte, Gorgas came and examined Jesse and stood by his bed. But there was nothing he could do. There was albumin in Jesse's urine, and then his kidneys shut down. Agramonte stood by the bed and looked at his friend. Jesse stared back from dark, sunken, delirious, dying eyes.

At the end he heaved and pitched, his body convulsing madly as the disease touched his brain and enveloped it. Early in the morning of September 25, 1900, two orderlies had to be summoned to hold him down. When the convulsions stopped they closed his eyes, expertly tied his wrists and ankles together, and removed the body. The bed was urgently needed.

*   *   *

When a soldier dies the Army collects his personal belongings and sends them to his next of kin. In this case the duty fell to Lieutenant Truby, the man who had developed the solar water heater.

As he methodically cataloged Jesse's possessions and packed them in a crate for delivery to Mabel, he discovered the notebook. He opened it, glanced through the first few pages, realized the implications, and started reading. As soon as he was finished, he sent an urgent message to Walter Reed in Washington.

Reed replied instantly, instructing Carroll to keep the notebook. A few days later, Reed was back in Havana.

As he read Lazear's notes, Reed's earlier skepticism about the mosquito theory vanished.

As Jesse had intended, his notes left no doubt. There was an infectious three-day period at the onset of yellow fever, and during that time it could be picked up by the house mosquito. Ten days later, the mosquito could transmit the disease, and perhaps a week later the next victim developed a fever. The agent still wasn't identified (viruses wouldn't appear in electron microscope viewscreens for decades yet), but if the vector was known, control of the disease was within grasp.

But Lazear's findings, no matter how convincing, were what scientists call preliminary. Confirming data was needed, and Reed launched a major experimental program, using volunteers, to accumulate enough data so that a paper could be published.

Reed, of course, was listed as first author of the paper. After all, hadn't he done most of the experiments? Lazear was mentioned, but got lesser billing. Carlos Finlay wasn't referred to at all.

Though Jesse's other belongings were sent to Mabel, Reed kept the little brown notebook when he returned to the United States. He was greeted as a hero. Later, while in his possession, the brown notebook mysteriously disappeared.

History credits Walter Reed with piecing together the yellow-fever puzzle, and a new Army medical center, which was to become one of the world's most prestigious research institutions, was named in his honor. Carroll, his assistant, is remembered for his loyalty and courage.

Gorgas, whose war against fomites had failed to quell yellow fever in Havana, was later sent to Panama. There he mounted one of the most massive mosquito-control campaigns in history, and all but eliminated yellow fever from the Canal Zone. In Panama, statues memorialize his accomplishment, which allowed the United States to succeed where France had failed.

But as for Jesse Lazear, he is often omitted from history books. His country built him no statues, and no hospital bears his name.

A BRAVE BUT TARNISHED
PRUSSIAN

Werner Forssmann was born in 1904, an auspicious year
that foreshadowed the new century. In New York, a
woman was arrested for smoking a cigarette in public. In
England, Rutherford and Soddy postulated the general
theory of radioactivity. In the Panama Canal Zone, work
began on the greatest engineering project since the Cheops
pyramid. Even Werner's own father, an earnest and hard-
working German, plied a trade that would come to epitomize the modern era: He sold policies for the Victoria Life
Insurance Company.

But the Berlin of Werner's childhood was the center of a
culture that looked back, not forward, one that refused to
embrace the future on its own terms and that dreamed,
instead, of imposing the past on it.

One of his earliest memories was of moving through a
dense and noisy crowd, gripping his father's strong and
familiar hand. Banners waved overhead, whipping and
cracking in the winter wind, and the music of a band rose
in the distance. Finally his father picked him up and balanced him on his shoulders. Werner clung desperately to
his perch, shrieking in fear and excitement.

From his vantage point he could see the broad cob-
blestone expanse of Unter den Linden, sparkling with

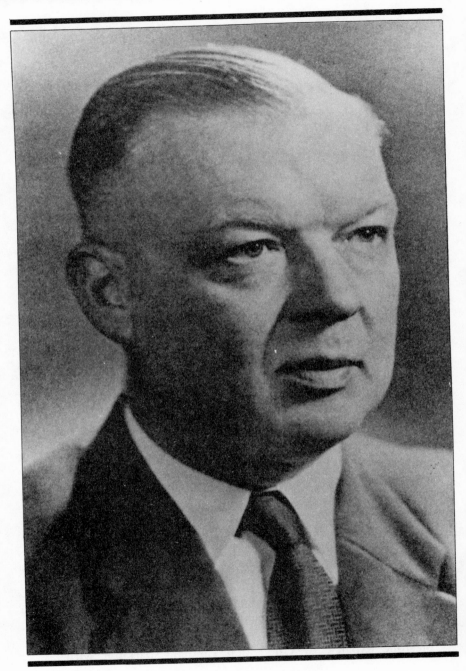

DR. WERNER FORSSMANN

frost. Friendly, fat policemen in blue uniforms, with long cavalry sabres at their waists and icicles in their moustaches, kept the crowd on the sidewalks.

Everyone carried a flag. Many of them were black and red, honoring the colors of the kaiser on this, his birthday, but there were also flags representing the individual federal states. Long banners hung from the roofs of the big stores, reaching almost to the ground. Frankfurter venders screamed above the din of talk and laughter.

The parade was led by the Army wagons, great clattering vehicles pulled by teams of huge, snorting horses whose muscles swelled and writhed just beneath their skins. Then came a prancing squadron of mounted policemen in dress uniform, followed by the Gardes du Corps. They had fierce, proud faces, many with dueling scars on their cheeks, and their uniforms glinted with polished silver and brass.

Breathlessly, Werner clutched his father's hair, his eyes glued on the mounted kettle drummer who followed at a proper distance. As he rolled the drum he periodically tossed his drumsticks high into the air, catching them expertly as they fell, never missing a beat. Behind the kettle drummer and a bearer of the royal banner came eight prancing chargers, carrying the emperor and his seven children. Excitement surged through the crowd and little Werner shrieked with the rest of them.

The emperor's birthday parade always took an hour and a half, and was followed by a general celebration that left young Werner overfed and exhausted. As his father put on his reserve officer's uniform and left for a regimental dinner, Werner was always put to bed. But sometimes he was awake, many hours later, when a noisy carriageful of men dropped his father at the front doorstep. It sometimes took his father several tries before he successfully replaced his sabre in the umbrella stand.

As Werner grew older he always remembered the emperor's birthdays with fondness, but some details clung to his mind more tenaciously than others. He never forgot the sight of Princess Viktoria-Luise riding sidesaddle, wearing the cape of her hussars and with a calpac perched on her head. Or that the emperor had a moustache exactly like his father's.

Werner's young eyes had also noted, and his juvenile mind recorded, an interesting fact about the kettle drummer. Though the man had tossed his drumsticks in the air with an air of confident precision, he apparently wasn't as perfect as he was supposed to appear. As he passed, young Werner had spied several spare drumsticks tucked into his polished black riding boot.

Werner's father, too, was a prudent man. He was as loyal as the next citizen, and loved Germany as much, but he wasn't subject to every emotion of the mob. He couldn't share the blind German animosity toward the French, for instance, and so Werner grew up without owning the toy soldiers and guns that the other children played with incessantly. When World War I began, his father donned his reserve uniform and left for the front, as he was ordered to do, but he departed with much fear and no enthusiasm. Werner never saw him again. ·

So Werner's formative years left him with a sense of grandeur, but not victory. With his father dead in the war and his mother growing bitter, with the hope-crushing hardship brought on by defeat and reparations, with Germany caught in an economic situation that presaged the Depression, Werner had special need of the desperately heroic dreams that make adolescence bearable.

He would never be a soldier, of course. He could never kill another human being, but there were other ways to be bold—better ways. In Werner's mind a surgeon was as intrepid as a soldier. Even an internist was, in his own way, an honorable force to be reckoned with. Perhaps Werner could one day be a doctor and make the life of his mother, and his fellowman, somehow better.

As he progressed toward the age of majority, the ambition became stronger and more refined. In 1922, straight from high school, he entered Friedrich Wilhelm University in Berlin.

At the medical school, science uneasily co-existed with a gestating new politic. Many of Werner's fellow students had been soldiers, and they were older and infinitely more experienced than he. Their minds were clouded with bitterness over the outcome of the war and dreams of future victories, and Werner often did better in his studies than they, but he understood that they needed their dreams. He had his own. His fantasy about operating on the heart, the most dramatic and mysterious organ of all, made the work go easier.

As a result, whenever his studies touched on the heart, he came to rapt attention. He thought it was the most fascinating of organs, though he didn't share the older generation's perception of it as the seat of the soul. In truth it was a pump, but that detracted nothing from its mystery. It was in fact a double pump, and it was the strongest, and the most durable, and the most complex pump that could be imagined.

And, increasingly, it was a killer.

The rise in heart disease in the 20th century was already becoming apparent, and was being used by philosophers of science to epitomize one of medicine's most basic enigmas: Each success leads to a new problem. Public health programs, launched by the Bavarian Pettenkofer and carried out by men like Gorgas in Panama, had eradicated malaria, yellow fever, typhoid, cholera, and plague from the civilized world. Vaccinations prevented smallpox, diphtheria, and tetanus.

The citizens who didn't die of those diseases now lived on, and grew older, and the arteries that fed their heart muscles became hard and narrow. Eventually they were struck by massive chest pain and, sooner or later, in the midst of agony, they died. Heart disease had taken its place as the 20th century's most potent killer, the medical equivalent of evil, a disease awaiting a hero . . . a dreamer . . . maybe even a young man named Werner Forssmann.

Though as a medical student he was obliged to devote most of his mental energy to the memorization of technical detail and to understanding the theory that tied that detail together, he couldn't help but be acutely aware of the deteriorating economic and social environment around him. For one thing, some of his teachers laced their medical teaching with political indoctrination.

Professor Otto Lubarsch, for instance, frequently explained to his classes that the Jews were the chief enemies of Germany—a charge that was particularly effective since Lubarsch was himself a Jew who had renounced his religion. Another of Werner's professors was involved in the Ludendorff movement, an effort to oust both Christianity and Judaism in favor of Wotan, the powerful god who had led the ancient Germanic warriors to their legendary victories.

The university was a hotbed of such theories and ambitions, and Werner could sympathize with them. But for him, medicine was the battlefield. Medicine, and surgery . . . and the heart.

Methodically, he broke the problem down. The heart diseases of aging were the ultimate target, but they wouldn't be the place to start. They were too complex. The first surgical campaign would probably be an attack on mechanical defects like congenital holes between the two sides of the heart. Something might even be done about scarred valves. But the surgeon looking for a bridgehead into the heart would do well to be conservative, to pick a simple problem, something that gave him a prayer of success. He would have to have the right equipment and . . .

The problem with dreams is that they progress in splendid leaps, whereas reality, pedestrian reality—reality crawls forward on trivia.

Werner could dream of operating on the heart, as other young doctors did, but in reality his best professors couldn't even make a proper diagnosis. An X ray could provide a hazy outline of the exterior of the heart, but gave the physician few clues as to what was going on inside. At many hospitals, electrical impulses from the heart were being recorded, but interpreting the squiggly lines that resulted was much like reading tea leaves.

In clinic, Werner and his fellow students were taught to make judgments about the heart based on sound. With a stethoscope you listened to heartbeats and heard, if you could, the tiny variations that indicated, say, a sticking valve. If you wanted to know if the heart was enlarged, you cocked your ear, like so, and you thumped the chest, just right, and you frowned and consulted the gods, and you made your diagnosis. It was all very mysterious and subjective, and either you were good at it or you weren't.

Werner wasn't, but his frustrations were tempered by his professors in anatomy and pathology. They said the best of clinicians misdiagnosed the heart as often as not. A definitive diagnosis could only be made at autopsy.

At autopsy! That was a bit late! How could you sew up holes in the heart if you couldn't even tell beforehand who had them and who didn't? Before heart surgery could become anything but a dream, the diagnosis problem would have to be solved.

But it was not, on reflection, a very difficult problem. The answer was almost intuitive and the techniques required had already been mastered by specialists in urology.

Urology, because of its focus on organs of excretion, has a humble reputation among laymen. But while the production and elimination of urine may not be a topic for polite conversation, it was a matter of life, death, and agony in the hospital. Kidney disease, if not corrected, was fatal. Elderly patients, especially men, suffered horribly when their prostates swelled sufficiently to block the flow from bladder to penis. In responding to these patients, the science of urology had leaped ahead of other disciplines.

As a medical student, Werner's exposure to urologic techniques centered around the relatively simple process of bladder catheterization. Because it often had to be done on an emergency basis at night and on weekends, catheterization was something the would-be doctors performed often.

The urethral catheter was a soft piece of rubber tubing about eighteen inches long and as thick as a pencil. It had a rounded end, with holes in either side. After scrubbing the pubic area and putting on sterile gloves, Werner grasped the penis in one hand and the lubricated tube in the other, placed the tube against the opening in the penis, and pushed gently but firmly.

The procedure had its dangers. For one thing, there is a sphincter muscle where the urethra opens into the bladder. That is the muscle that controls urination, and it isn't entirely voluntary. If the medical student pushed too hard, and the catheter traumatized the sphincter, it might clamp down. Then the rubber catheter couldn't be forced in at all and a steel one would have to be used.

But like many medical fallback positions, that one was dangerous. Make one wrong move with a steel-tipped catheter and you would poke a hole in the wall of the urinary tract. Then germs would get in from other parts of the body, contaminate the urinary tract, climb to the kidneys, and kill the patient. No, it was better to do it correctly in the first place, with the rubber catheter.

Catheterization required and deserved the student's deepest concentration.

But running a tube up into the bladder was simple compared to the process that had been developed to traverse the narrow ureters that run from the bladder up to the kidneys themselves. Kidney catheterization was the most sophisticated diagnostic procedure in all of medicine and the medical students, while not allowed to participate, were encouraged to watch.

The process began with the insertion of a cystoscope, a hollow rod incorporating lights and lenses, into the bladder. Then, squinting into the instrument and maneuvering the lenses and lights on the far end, the urologist located the two holes that led upward to the kidneys.

Once the holes were located, an assistant broke out twenty-five- to forty-inch-long ureteral catheters. Peering into the eyepieces, taking it painfully slowly, the urologist threaded the catheters up through the tube of the cystoscope into the bladder, and from there, carefully, carefully, maneuvered them into the ureters and up to the kidneys.

With the tubes in the kidneys, many things became possible. Samples of urine could be gathered for analysis, and doctors could tell which kidney was causing problems. Contrast medium that was opaque to X rays could be injected into the kidney, and radiographic pictures could outline the interior of the organ and reveal any structural malformations.

In the same way, Werner reasoned, a tube in the heart would allow physicians to take pressure readings inside the great pump itself, and could be used to inject dyes and contrast mediums. The result should be X-ray photographs of the inside of the heart, photographs capable of revealing mechanical defects such as congenital holes, crossed vessels, and diseased valves.

It wasn't an original idea. A few hours in the library

revealed to Werner that as long ago as the 1860s a pair of Frenchmen had successfully introduced catheters into the hearts of horses. Their reports were complete with old-fashioned illustrations.

One picture in particular attracted the young man's attention. It was a drawing of a man standing beside a horse. The man was holding a tube that appeared to be as thick as a man's finger. One end of the tube was connected to an apparatus, and the other end disappeared into the jugular vein in the horse's neck. A cutaway drawing of the interior of the animal's chest showed a small, inflated rubber balloon inside the horse's right ventricle.

According to the text, the beating of the heart put pressure on the balloon. The pressure was transferred via the tube to the apparatus, where it was converted to a graph that recorded the up and down, up and down, up and down pressures of the beating heart. Werner was fascinated. What a wonderful, elegant, bold experiment. He stared at the picture, mesmerized, and it burned itself into his mind.

So his idea wasn't even new. But it had not, as far as Werner could determine, ever been applied to humans.

At the time, immersed as he was in medical school, Werner's thoughts on heart disease diagnosis were hurried and incomplete. Most of his energies were devoted to study and to the educational drudgery of clinical chores. In the summertime he worked as an assistant to a physician. There were always snatches of time for dreams, but never enough time to do anything about them.

As one hectic day followed another and graduation approached, there was the added pressure of finding a job in the depressed German economy. Things were so bad that some of his wealthier classmates had volunteered their services, without salary, in order to get accepted for further training at a decent hospital. Werner, who was anything but rich, was deeply grateful when a friend, whose father's illness prevented him from taking an assignment at a women's hospital in Spandau, passed along the job to Werner. It was a humble position, but it was better than nothing. At least, that was what he thought at the time.

At Spandau, however, his determination dwindled in the face of interminable scut work. He was expected to see the women at clinic, but had to pass the interesting cases along to senior physicians. He was obligated to make house calls, several each day, to women dying of pelvic infections—and for whom he could do little or nothing. And, worst of all, he was responsible for heat therapy treatments.

Heat therapy for vaginal inflammation was the big money-maker for the clinic, and for four or five hours each day Werner was required to operate the control panel.

As he sat at the panel, in the middle of the treatment room, the ladies of Spandau arrived at the clinic four at a time. Each took her place in one of the room's four screened-off corners, where she disrobed and applied the heating element to her private parts. For the following half hour Werner sat at the control panel, bored beyond belief, watching the dials and wishing desperately to be someplace else. When the half hour was finished he gave a signal and the four women dressed and scuttled out, to be replaced by four more. Within a month of Werner's grateful acceptance of the job, he was looking furiously for another, anything, anywhere, quickly.

Suddenly, his luck seemed to change. Worried by the desperation she saw in her son's letters, his mother spoke to a friend whose older brother, a certain Dr. Richard Schneider, was chief of one of the surgical departments in the Auguste Viktoria Home, a Red Cross hospital in Eberswalde. A few days later Werner was talking on the telephone to Dr. Schneider, trying to keep the urgency out of his voice as he answered, yes, sir; no, sir; of course, sir; he could be available as soon as he could get his bags packed, sir.

In Eberswalde, everything was different. Dr. Schneider was a kind man and he immediately took a shine to the sincere and enthusiastic young doctor who learned surgery so quickly. For a while he listened indulgently as Werner showed up in his office time and time again, enthusiastic about some new, complicated operation he had just learned to perform.

Finally, though, Dr. Schneider's duties as a teacher led him to interrupt his brash young student and instruct him, gently but firmly, that there were no such things as "complicated operations." There were only clumsy surgeons. Embarrassed and chagrined, Werner stopped boasting.

Though his work was hard and his hours were long, Werner could sense that his education was progressing rapidly, and he loved his new job. After escaping from a seemingly endless stream of matrons with swollen vaginas, a surgical internship at Eberswalde was paradise.

He worked alongside another young man, Dr. Peter Romeis, and the shared pressure quickly led to comradeship. Peter, too, had thought about the heart problem and was hungry to work on the frontier. What was more, he liked Werner's idea of putting a catheter into the heart and releasing some X-ray-opaque material.

Obviously, though, you couldn't enter the jugular vein in a human—not to merely make a diagnosis, in any event. Opening the jugular vein in a human was a messy business and it would leave a hideous scar. As a practical matter, the entry point for the catheter should probably be the big vein in the inside of the elbow, the same convenient one that was used for most intravenous injections.

They decided that if they inserted the catheter into the arm and held the arm out by the patient's side, they would have a straight run at the heart. The catheter should slide naturally into the subclavian vein, and from there into the vena cava, and finally into the right atrium, the entry chamber in the right side of the heart. When they were satisfied with their plan, they approached Dr. Schneider.

Dr. Schneider listened indulgently as his young assistants explained how it would be done. The vein in the arm would be opened, and a ureteral catheter would be inserted into the heart. It was simple, they said. Foolproof. An injection of novocaine into the skin over the vein incision would be the only anesthetic necessary, though a tranquilizer would probably help make the patient calmer.

The surgical chief sat back in his chair, considering the proposition thoughtfully. Finally he agreed, almost reluctantly, that the world needed a better way to visualize the inside of the living heart. And Werner's idea just might be the way to do it, but . . .

The problem was . . .

Science was a wonderful thing, that was not to be denied, but there were realities in life. . . .

The problem was that the Red Cross hospital wasn't like a medical school, exactly. The demand was for quality, true, but the daily surgical schedule dealt more often with hemorrhoids, gallbladders, and cesarean births.

What if they tried it on a patient and the patient died?

What would happen was that Dr. Schneider would inevitably be summoned and asked to explain why the chief of surgery, in an unsophisticated little hospital out in the countryside—the word "provincial" would undoubtedly be used—why such a doctor was encouraging his interns to go around sticking things into his patients' hearts. It would be a difficult question to answer.

Well, the young men argued, the problem wouldn't arise. The patient wouldn't die.

Dr. Schneider thought a moment. Perhaps. Perhaps. First . . . they should do some animal experiments. . . . Yes . . . animal experiments were definitely called for. Why didn't they go and do some animal experiments?

Misunderstanding the olive branch, Werner brushed the suggestion aside. No, sir. Animal experiments had been conducted over a period of seventy years, and nothing had ever happened to the animals. He had the references with him. The proposed experiment was safe. There was a reason to do it, to make way for heart surgery. It should be done. It needed to be done.

Perhaps, Dr. Schneider finally conceded. But not at his hospital.

No, said Dr. Schneider firmly.

. . . but . . .

No!

Werner thought about it for a moment and then tried another tack. Dr. Schneider's objection, if he understood it correctly, had to do with the risk to the patient. Well, there was another approach.

"I'll do it on myself, then," said Werner.

Dr. Schneider looked speculatively at the young man. Finally he took a deep breath and shook his head.

"My dear Dr. Forssmann," he said, addressing Werner with an unusual formality, "I'm afraid I must also forbid that. . . . Don't look at me so reproachfully!"

The old man's face became firm, and his tone of voice left no room for argument.

"I know you're going to say you can do whatever you like with your own body, but there are limits to that, too. Remember your mother. I am also responsible to her for what you do. Imagine how it would be if I had to inform this lady, who's already lost her husband in the war, that her only son had died in my hospital as a result of an experiment which I had approved. Put yourself in my position! In any case, you may be sure that my no is final and absolute."

Chastized, Werner left the chief surgeon's office. There was no doubt in his mind that Dr. Schneider was mistaken but, mistaken or not, he remained the chief of surgery, and authority was authority. . . .

On the other hand, authority could be wrong. Hadn't even the kaiser been wrong, in his war with France? How many died for that error? And how many would die, unnecessarily, if the medical profession didn't proceed with all reasonable haste toward the age of heart surgery?

So the question wasn't really whether or not to disobey Dr. Schneider. The question was how Werner could get his hands on the proper equipment without arousing suspicion. He needed help from someone with access to sterile surgical equipment.

Werner thought over the problem for several days before settling on Gerda Ditzen. She was the chief surgical nurse, and while she could be as commanding as a headwaiter, she could also be a soft touch for a handsome young surgeon. Furthermore, since she and Werner had on occasion lent one another books, the ice was already broken.

She wasn't stupid, though, so the game had to be subtle. In his own words, he started "to prowl around Gerda like a sweet-toothed cat around a cream jug."

The ideal time for the experiment, Werner figured, would be right after lunch. The German culture, like the Spanish, provides for a siesta . . . so everyone would be napping and the operating room areas would be clear. Werner began to dawdle in the canteen after eating, hoping to meet Nurse Gerda as she left the nurses' dining room.

He made the encounters seem, to her, like chance meetings. They shared a joke and a little gossip, and it was natural for her to invite Werner back to her little office next to the operating room, where her rank entitled her to keep a coffeepot. Cautiously, Werner steered the conversation from gossip to ambition, from ambition to dream, from dream to heart surgery, from heart surgery to the problem of diagnosis.

Gerda listened politely at first, then became intrigued. It wasn't often that a doctor solicited her opinion on such things, and she borrowed several of Werner's books. She was flattered by his straightforward assumption that she would understand them.

And of course, he was absolutely right. He was right that she could master the technical articles, and he was right in theory at least that the experiment he proposed would be perfectly safe. On the other hand, she knew from years in the operating room that there was a huge difference between theory and reality, and a man was a more delicate creature than a horse. Still, a man wasn't *that* much more delicate. . . . No . . . it should be safe, and it would mean so much to young Werner, and maybe . . . maybe even to the world.

But, she reminded herself, as long as the chief of surgery forbade the experiment, her judgment was academic. If Werner did it anyway (and she could tell he was tempted), it would probably ruin his career. The situation was ironic. It was safe, of that she was growing increasingly certain—safe, except that it was capable of destroying Werner professionally.

But it would be such a grand experiment!

One day, about two weeks after Schneider had told Werner to forget it, she sighed aloud to him, "What a pity that we can't do the experiment together."

Werner struggled to keep his composure. That evening he thought it through.

Nurse Gerda, he decided, was ripe.

The next day was a beautiful one, an early summer day with a clear blue sky and daisies blooming in the flower-beds of the city, a day of nesting birds and playing children. The morning passed slowly. Lunch tasted like sawdust. He watched from a distance, seemingly engrossed in a book, as Nurse Gerda returned to her cubicle. Then he carefully closed the book and rose to his feet. The moment had come.

Nurse Gerda was pleased to see Werner enter her office, but her smile changed to a baffled expression as he started giving her orders in the imperious tone of a surgeon. He said he wanted the equipment required to open a vein under sterile conditions. He also wanted a sterile ureteral catheter, one of the long ones designed to go from the bladder to the kidney.

Her head spun. Did he think she was a fool? Or afraid of him?

She laid her book aside carefully, but kept her seat. She wasn't aware, she said, that anyone on the ward was scheduled for a venesection. Besides, why a ureteral catheter?

She looked him square in the eyes. "You're not planning to do that experiment of yours against the boss's orders, are you?"

Werner beamed back at her. "Nurse Gerda, you need know nothing about what I'm going to do. But supposing I was to do the experiment—it would be quite safe."

She eyed him closely. "Are you absolutely sure there's no danger?"

Absolutely.

Nurse Gerda thought about it for a minute. "All right then," she finally said. "Do it to me. I put myself in your hands."

Werner's smile vanished. This was a possibility he hadn't anticipated. Should he accept her offer? Was the experiment really safe, perfectly safe? He was willing to try it on a patient, even on himself. But Nurse Gerda was so trusting, so, almost, innocent, and he had taken shameless advantage of her. His mind raced. Career. Mankind. Curiosity.

"Well . . ." He stalled for a moment, looking away from her. Then his face relaxed.

". . . well . . . why not? You'll be the first person in history to undergo such an experiment."

She rose from her chair and headed toward the supply room. Werner followed her there, and then to the operating room. After the equipment was ready, she sat down and extended her arm, baring the inside of her elbow. Werner stood above her, apparently lost in thought.

It would be better, Werner finally suggested in a businesslike voice, if she would lie down on the operating table.

She looked at him and at the table. She frowned slightly, hesitating.

Werner's heart raced. Quickly, before she could think, he reminded her that a shot of novocaine will make an occasional patient faint, and he would have to give her novocaine where he was going to open her vein. She didn't want to ruin the experiment by banging her head on the floor, did she?

Nurse Gerda considered the explanation, accepted it. She climbed up onto the table, wriggled a little to find a comfortable position, and again extended her arm.

Quickly, Werner reached under the table for the leather strap used to pin the patient's legs. It was around the nurse's knees and tightly buckled before she could protest. She sat up, swearing at Werner and trying to free herself. But at her age she was no longer limber enough to reach the buckle without bending her knees.

Werner soothed her. It was just another precaution against her fainting, he said. After all, he didn't want her rolling off the table.

Suspicious, but having no practical means of objecting, she lay back on the table and, once again, extended her arm. She could hear Werner adjusting the instrument tray just above her head. She tried to twist her head upward to see what he was doing, but her neck wouldn't arch that far.

He stood behind her, watching her carefully as he silently slid the novocaine needle into his own flesh. Ignoring the stinging pain, he sent the needle darting here and there under the skin, pressing the plunger firmly, numbing as large an area as he could as rapidly as possible.

Then, to give the novocaine time to take effect, he bent over Nurse Gerda's elbow and made a big production of preparing it, scrubbing the skin first with iodine and then with alcohol and finally laying a sterile cloth over it. She seemed reassured that he was being so careful.

As he stepped back out of her view she closed her eyes and relaxed her arm, preparing for the coming prick of the needle. She could hear him fumbling with the equipment again.

Behind her head Werner worked furiously, slitting the skin, finding the vein, and opening it. Blood dripped down his arm and onto the floor, but he paid no attention to it. The catheter tip went into the vein easily, and he snaked it about a foot up. Then he coiled up the remaining length of catheter and pressed a wad of sterile cotton over the point where it entered the skin. He stepped back into Nurse Gerda's view. With his catheterized arm crooked over the coil, he had his other arm free to quickly unsnap the strap.

"There we are," he said, smiling. "It's ready now. Please call the X-ray nurse."

It took a moment for Nurse Gerda to understand what had been done. Then she sat bolt upright on the table, yelling curses at him. Suddenly she shut up.

He was a doctor. There was a crisis. He was giving her orders.

X ray.

They needed to get ready down in X ray.

Obediently, she leaped off the table and ran for the telephone.

By the time they arrived downstairs, the chief X-ray nurse had the fluoroscope ready and Werner stepped behind the screen. He strained to bend his body so that he could see his own chest through the screen, but he couldn't bend his neck enough. He needed a mirror.

Nurse Gerda disappeared to fetch one. The X-ray nurse stood where she was, trying to understand what was going on. When she did, she turned and disappeared.

When Nurse Gerda returned with a hand mirror, Werner held it on the other side of the screen, tilting it this way and that as he examined the image. It was perfect. Absolutely perfect. The catheter showed up beautifully, extending up his left arm all the way to shadows that marked the boundary of his chest. He propped the mirror in place; eyes fixed on it, he held up his left arm and, with his right, prepared to push the catheter home.

His concentration was interrupted when, at that moment, the door flew open and Peter Romeis burst in. His eyes were sleepy and his hair was tousled, but he was fully awake.

"You idiot," he screamed, lunging for Werner's left arm in an attempt to pull out the catheter, "what the hell are you doing?"

Werner stepped deftly aside, kicking Peter sharply in the shin.

As Peter collapsed in the corner, howling in pain, Werner stepped back to the fluoroscope. Again focusing his eyes on the mirror, he extended his left arm. With his right hand he grasped the remaining length of catheter and, gently but firmly, pushed.

In the fluoroscope, the catheter's shadow moved an inch into the chest. Werner pushed again, and again the shadow penetrated deeper. Slowly, in inch-long leaps, it moved toward the beating shape of the heart, touched it, moved farther, and finally stopped, its tip in the first of the heart's four chambers. There it hesitated, then moved again, deeper into the writhing shadow, until it reached the center of what Werner took to be the right ventricle.

Peter, who by now had stopped moaning, pulled himself to his feet and limped around to the front of the fluoroscope screen. He warned Werner to take it out, but Werner stepped behind an X-ray machine, ignoring him. There was the ka-*chunk* of relays closing, followed by the sound of plates being changed. Ka-*chunk*, ka-*chunk*, ka-*chunk*. In the background, the telephone was ringing.

Finally, certain that he had taken enough X rays to document what he had done, Werner removed the catheter. He let Peter dress the wound.

That was the switchboard on the telephone, Peter said as he closed the incision. As might be expected Dr. Schneider was waiting to see Werner, in his office, immediately.

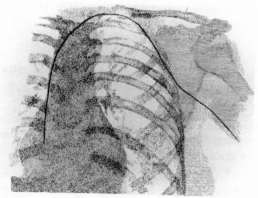

The X ray of Forssmann's chest that documented the insertion of the catheter in a vein of his left arm, extending into his heart

From The History of Cardiac Surgery *by Stephen L. Johnson, courtesy Johns Hopkins University Press, Baltimore*

For the first time, Werner felt a twinge of fear. He brushed it aside. After all, the experiment had succeeded!

But by the time he got to the chief's office his confidence, along with the novocaine, was wearing off. Facing the old man's icy anger, Werner's success seemed minor . . . compared to the breach of faith. Standing in front of Dr. Schneider's desk, he stammered out a defense—but now, for some reason, it sounded feeble and shabby. Miserably, he heard himself apologizing.

Dr. Schneider sat, impassive, his eyes fixed on the favored young man who had betrayed his trust. When the door opened and a technician appeared, he reached out his hand for the sheaf of X-ray films. He let Werner stand there as he held each film up to the light and examined it carefully.

The young man had been right, of course. And Dr. Schneider did like him. And since Werner would pay the price, he should have the credit that was due him. The old surgeon let his face relax.

Finally he turned to Werner, smiled, and extended his hand. "Forssmann, you've made a great discovery, and I must congratulate you. . . ."

Werner was confused by the change of attitude. Suddenly the old man seemed genuinely pleased that Werner had made a discovery . . . but, at the same time, Werner had to understand, he wasn't exactly fired, but neither could he stay.

"I believe you and your ideas are out of place now in my little provincial hospital. You should be somewhere where you'll have more scope to carry out your plans. I'll do everything in my power to help you . . . but . . . first we must celebrate."

News of the experiment quickly made the rounds of the hospital, and the festivities were well attended and noisy.

Again and again Werner was toasted. The young man had never before in his life been made to feel so important.

Dr. Schneider's anger never again surfaced, and Werner forgot it. The next day, and during the days following, Werner met frequently with the chief of surgery to discuss the paper that was to be submitted on the experiment.

In the meantime, Dr. Schneider called a number of his contacts in the surgical world and, before long, found Werner a position at Charité Hospital in Berlin. There he would work under the famous Dr. Ferdinand Sauerbruch.

It was nothing like being fired. When the time came for Werner to leave, Dr. Schneider seemed genuinely sad to see him go. As he grasped the young man's hand he even seemed to be trying to offer some fatherly advice, to warn him, almost, trying to tell him something about the way the world was. But Werner, intent on the future and his career, didn't listen. He dreamed, instead, of the lecture-ship that would soon be his, once the paper on cardiac catheterization was published.

In Berlin, Werner strolled into the Charité Hospital and Dr. Sauerbruch's office as though he belonged there. Dr. Sauerbruch greeted him warmly, but he judged immediately that the new man was wanting in discipline, not to mention respect. In Dr. Sauerbruch's mind, instilling that respect was one of the most important functions of a teacher.

Werner soon learned, in various unsubtle ways, that he was expected to conduct himself more humbly in the presence of senior doctors, and particularly Dr. Sauerbruch. He was to do as he was told, his immediate superiors instructed him, and he was never, never to contradict his seniors. Independent thought was frowned on among students. . . . There would be time for that later, much later. Go along, his fellow junior doctors advised him, and he would get along.

It wasn't so bad, they said, once you got used to it.

Werner was appalled. If you were a sycophant in your formative years, how would you become anything different later? And to think that he, with an important paper in press already . . . and his work wasn't only in a scientific journal, but in a popular magazine as well! And they wanted him to crawl!

The surgeons at Charité saw it differently. To them he was a sensation seeker. A journal article wasn't good enough for him; he had to go to the popular press as well! Werner denied it, but wasn't believed. One senior surgeon stopped him in the hallway, brandishing the journal paper.

"This is a fine kettle of fish," the man snarled, "but you won't get away with tricks like that in our department!"

A general dislike for Werner grew rapidly among the members of the Charité surgical staff and spread to the students and the nursing staff. Everywhere he turned, he found hostility. He responded in kind.

Finally, confused but insistent, he confronted Dr. Sauerbruch regarding his lectureship.

Dr. Sauerbruch looked at Werner with none of Dr. Schneider's generosity. "You might lecture in a circus with your little tricks," he retorted, "but never in a German university."

As 1929 ended, the entire world having followed Germany into its depression, Werner Forssmann was without a job. The forever tolerant Dr. Schneider took him back temporarily, smoothed things over with Dr. Sauerbruch, and, in a few months, sent the young man back to Charité. This time Werner was much humbler, and he lasted almost eighteen months before Dr. Sauerbruch booted him out again.

Vaguely, proudly, refusing to bend to the whims of inferior intellects, Werner struggled to weather the emotional storm. He perceived that the world was somehow out of step, and that made him a misfit, and—like many other misfits in Germany—he began to yearn for the old to be born anew.

Werner came to believe, like Adolf Hitler, that there was something essentially fine and brave about Germany and that, by extension, and despite everything, there was also something fine and brave about himself.

And if the fatherland was in difficult times, so was he. The blame focused on political miasmas . . . on ill-defined evil forces, outside influences. Perhaps his teachers at college had been correct in their accusations against the Jews. The year he lost his position at Charité for the second and final time, Werner joined the Nazi party. It was an act for which most of his colleagues in other countries would never forgive him.

He found a job at a hospital in Mainz, on the condition that he remain single. The following year, he married.

He landed another job, not a very good one, in Berlin's Rudolf Virchow Hospital. Because he had had some experience with catheters, he was assigned to urology. He hated it, and moved to a surgical job in Dresden . . . but they didn't pay him what he was worth, and there was a falling-out. He found another position at the Robert Koch Hospital in Berlin, but they didn't appreciate him there, either. . . .

At least, once again, there were parades in the street. Once again the people waved flags as the boots of the soldiers struck the paving in unison, loudly, the clump, clump, clump of their goosestepping rising above the shrieks of the admiring crowds. By the time the war began, Werner was already in the Army.

The next years passed, first in glorious victory and later in desperate, bloody battle. Werner served on first the Polish and then the Norwegian front, then was transferred south again for the disastrous campaign against the Russians. Finally he fled, with the rest of the German Army, before the advancing Soviet troops.

He swam the Elbe River to reach American-occupied territory, and eventually was reunited with his wife in the Black Forest.

Perhaps, by this time, he had given up his dream. He still talked about heart surgery, but without the old certainty that it would ever happen. He hadn't seen a medical journal since the war began, and the priority now was survival, reconstruction, the preservation of what little hadn't been destroyed.

Doctors were needed desperately, so Werner opened a private practice, and soon his office was full of patients. They had little they could pay with, but they appreciated what he did and for the first time he had a sense of peace, of belonging, of being accepted.

Occasionally the outer world intruded. A Swiss emissary arrived at his door, asking for Dr. Werner Forssmann. *The* Dr. Werner Forssmann, the first man to catheterize a human heart. Would he come to Switzerland to be honored?

Werner and his wife were dumbfounded to learn that during the long war, while Werner treated wounded soldiers, surgeons all over the world had taken up his dream of heart surgery. Now they were routinely snaking catheters into people's hearts, sampling blood, and injecting contrast medium. Rapid-fire X-ray machines allowed moving pictures of the heart muscle to be made as the dye streamed through the arteries, revealing which were clear and which were blocked. There was confidence that heart surgery would soon become possible.

Any serious student of the subject could find out, by consulting his medical library, that the seminal paper on heart catheterization had been written in 1929 by one W. Forssmann, an intrepid young intern who disobeyed his superiors and ran a ureteral catheter into his own heart. To a small group of people, Werner was famous.

But Werner, gripped in the confines of war, had known nothing of this. And now he was a physician, a happy and prosperous man, gracefully growing old in the Black Forest. He took the honors in stride and ignored them.

But on August 18, 1956, his peace was shattered forever. There was no ignoring the telegram from Stockholm informing him that he had won the Nobel Prize.

Suddenly there were reporters on the telephone and others camped on his front lawn, hungry for more details of the daring young man who stuck a catheter into his own heart.

The reporters all mentioned, of course, that the story had a tragic side, and that the young man, weak in some way perhaps, was now an ex-Nazi.

Buffeted by the combination of praise and reproach, the fire returned to Werner's professional life. Turning his back on his practice, he applied to fill a vacancy as chief of surgery in a prominent hospital in Düsseldorf. As a Nobel laureate, he naturally got it.

But, Nobel or no Nobel, Werner was no longer a young man with a dream. He was now on the downside of middle age and the brashness had turned to stubbornness, the dreams to carping bitterness. If a patient died, it was someone else's fault. He repeatedly accused his fellow department heads of incompetence. He stalked out of meetings. He imagined he was being discussed surreptitiously, and he was correct. Meetings were being conducted about him.

It wasn't easy to fire a Nobel laureate but, given sufficient motive, neither was it impossible. After all, the man was clearly a misfit. And he had been, it had to be remembered, a Nazi. Soon Werner was back in the Black Forest, even bitterer than before, trying to pick up what was left of his practice.

Heart surgery, in the meantime, became possible. The patient was chilled ahead of time, giving the surgeon several minutes to stop the heart, reach in, and cut free a malformed valve. Scientists worked furiously on a heart-lung machine. As Werner always knew it would, chest surgery became the frontier.

But Werner, who had helped make the revolution possible, had no further role to play in it. He was left behind in the Black Forest, a misfit who deserved the credit he got but was a misfit nonetheless.

Like so many of his Nazi colleagues he devoted the last years of his life to composing an autobiography explaining how it had been that the world, and not Werner Forssmann, had been so badly out of step.

The world was no longer interested, of course, and the book sold poorly. Werner died in 1980.

A DANGEROUS TRANSFUSION

The relentless grind of medical school is largely composed of events and details that blend into one another as they fade into the past, yet there are always certain formative experiences that etch themselves forever into the student's mind. A psychiatrist may never forget when as a medical student he fumbled with the cage door of the dog he was assigned to operate on and saw the wretched creature wag its tail and lick his hand. A scientist may remember, to his death, the one splendid instant in which he was struck by a vivid insight into the nature of the bacteriological world. And for many a clinician there is a single patient who clings to the mind, nagging, aching, haunting.

For Bill Harrington she was seventeen, she was pretty, she was frightened, and, like himself, she was Boston Irish. He first saw her the day she was admitted to the charity ward.

It was her prettiness that struck him first, as he stepped through the wall of curtains that had been erected to protect her privacy. Her parents sat one on each side of the bed, and they stood up when Bill entered. The girl looked up at him with respect, fear, and hope.

In fact Bill was no doctor at all, merely a third-year medical student at nearby Tufts University. But it was

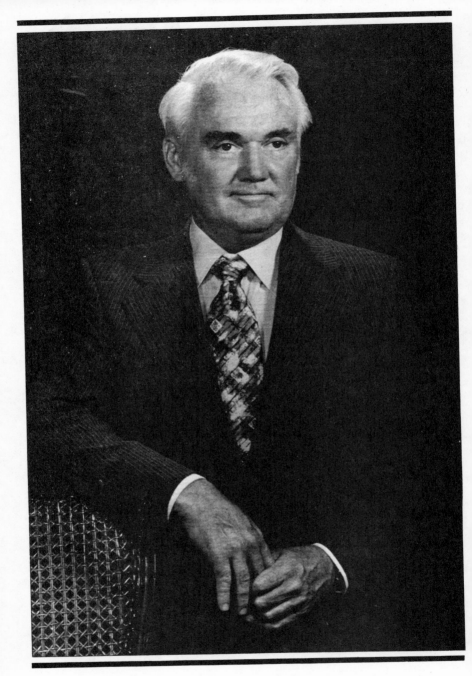

DR. WILLIAM J. HARRINGTON

Courtesy Dr. Harrington

1945 and, with most of the *real* doctors off to war, the hospitals were being staffed by the very old and the very young. Bill earned his room and board by spending nights and weekends at this particular hospital, where he did the scut work on charity patients and generally made himself useful. Of necessity he had what later generations of medical school students would consider to be broad powers over the lives of the Irish couple and their apprehensive daughter.

For an instant he stopped, his twenty-two-year-old mind frozen by the fact of the girl's prettiness, and then he moved into the curtain-enclosed space. He shook the father's strong, callused hand, nodded to the mother, and opened the metal cover of the girl's patient record. Taking a pencil from the pocket of his white jacket, he explained that he would have to get some information for the admissions form.

Bill sat with his clipboard balanced on his knee, asking his clipped, clinical questions and writing down the answers in detail. At first the girl looked directly at him, but when the questions turned intimate she blushed and lowered her eyes. She searched haltingly for the polite words for the things she needed to express. Bill tried to make it easier for her by remaining very professional, translating her embarrassed phrases into words like "hemorrhage" and "vagina." She had been experiencing heavy bleeding from the vagina for several days.

The medical student kept his face carefully impassive, though the shocking diagnosis was already forming in his mind: aborted pregnancy. Girls often came in with severe bleeding after seeing an abortionist, or after trying to abort themselves with knitting needles or pieces of wire. Sometimes they died. This patient's symptoms were consistent with that, and yet . . . he could not reconcile the diagnosis with the poignantly virginal patient in front of him.

Making himself appear casual, Bill raised his head and let his eyes brush across the scene, taking in the devoted mother, the embarrassed girl, and the worried father.

Bill said nothing to reveal his thoughts. He finished with his questions, snapped the book closed, and stood up. He would have to examine the patient now, he said, pressing the bedside call button. In a few moments a nurse appeared and ushered the parents outside the wall of curtains. Then the nurse returned. It was especially important, when the patient was so pretty, to have a nurse in the room.

Obediently, the girl sat up in bed and Bill bent close, shining a flashlight into each of her eyes. The pupils contracted normally. The whites of her eyes showed no touch of yellow jaundice. The nurse handed him a tongue depressor and the girl, as instructed, said, "Ah." There was no sign of inflammation. Her ears were healthy—and clean. His fingers probed the softness of her neck. If the bleeding wasn't caused by an abortion then it could be leukemia, but he failed to find the telltale enlarged lymph nodes. Then Bill stood aside as the nurse sat the girl up and untied the hospital gown.

The girl modestly clutched the gown at the shoulders as it fell apart to reveal her naked back. Bill made the clinical observation that her skin was as clear and white as the finest marble. He thumped on her back and was rewarded with a healthy, hollow sound. She gasped as the cold metal of the stethoscope touched her warm skin. She stared straight ahead as he slid his hand beneath her gown, reached under her arm, and rested his palm under her left breast, just over the apex of her racing heart. It was all very normal.

As Bill detailed this normality in the chart the nurse laid the girl down, pulled the blanket up beneath her gown to cover her pubis, and then pulled back the gown until it covered only her breasts. That left her midriff exposed.

"Just relax," he said, in what he hoped was a comforting voice. He stepped to the bedside and, as the nurse watched impassively, gently but firmly he massaged her belly while observing her face for any sign of pain. There was none. She stifled a giggle.

He pushed harder, probing in vain for tumor masses or indications of a tubal pregnancy. Her eyes widened as he pushed firmly under her rib cage, checking the size of her liver. The spleen didn't seem enlarged, either.

As Bill again stepped aside to write in the chart the nurse pulled the covers up under the girl's chin, and then adjusted the bedclothes to reveal her shapely right leg. With a rubber-tipped hammer Bill tapped her beneath her kneecap. Her leg jerked. He ran a finger lightly across the sole of her foot, and her big toe turned downward. The other limb behaved likewise. All normal.

As the nurse helped the girl retie her gown, Bill turned away and pushed through the curtains. He told the parents that they could return to the bedside, then walked down to the end of the ward to finish working on the chart at the nurses' station.

For fifteen minutes he stood, bent over the metal-clad record book, writing out his observations in great detail. He was puzzled, still unable to square his sense of the girl's modesty with the clinical evidence of an illegitimate pregnancy followed by a botched abortion. Yet he could think of nothing else it could be.

Finally he sighed, closed the chart, and placed it in the rack. He had other problems to attend to, like checking on the woman with heart failure and the old man who couldn't pass water. Before the night was over, Bill was certain, he would have to relieve the man's bladder with a catheter.

The next two hours passed, lost in the routine of work on the ward, with a few spare minutes in which to review his neuroanatomy notes for an upcoming quiz. Then it was time for rounds, and he found himself tiredly following an equally exhausted Ob-Gyn resident from bed to bed, checking on all the patients Bill had admitted that day.

Finally they stood before the pretty Irish girl. Her mother and father were still there.

The resident nodded a curt greeting in the direction of the patient and her parents, then opened the chart. His eyes rested for a moment on the Irish name, then glanced over the list of symptoms. In a moment he looked up.

"You've had an abortion," he said matter-of-factly.

The girl looked at him, an expression of surprise coming onto her face and then, as the implications sank home, crumbling into a stare of sheer horror.

"No," she said hollowly and then, louder, *"No!"*

She looked at her mother, but her mother's face had turned to stone. She turned to look at her father, hesitated, and averted her face. The resident had already turned away and was talking to the medical student about a blood work-up.

"No," the girl said again, much more softly now. "No."

Her father leaned toward the bed, placing his hand over hers. "Now, Peggy," he said gently, "now tell the truth."

"I *am* telling the truth," the girl burst out, then collapsed into sobs.

His instructions to Bill finished, the resident turned back toward the bed. The mother seemed to be in shock and the girl wasn't in any condition to listen, so the resident addressed his words to the father. His daughter would need an operation, tonight, to stop the bleeding. Either he or his wife would have to be on hand to sign the necessary permission forms.

That said, the resident turned and departed through the curtains. Bill hesitated. With an extreme force of will he squelched his churning emotions. He didn't have time for feelings. He had work to do. Finally he turned and followed the resident, the girl's sobs ringing in his ears.

The resident went to the clinical laboratory and picked up the telephone. As Bill assembled the equipment he needed for the presurgical blood studies, he heard the senior man order the telephone operator to page the surgical resident. A few minutes later Bill was back at the girl's bedside with the blood study tray.

The girl had composed herself now, though her eyes were red and puffy from crying. She obediently held out her left hand and looked away as Bill took the tip of her middle finger, squeezed it, and stabbed it with a pointed metal lancet. He sucked the resulting drop of blood into a thin glass tube, squeezed out another drop, and captured it in a second tube. A third drop ended up as a smear on a slide.

By the time Bill got to the laboratory the blood on the slide was dry and brown. He deposited a few drops of stain on it and looked at his watch. When one minute had passed he added some water to dilute the stain and then set the slide aside. He would allow ten minutes for the stain to set, then would rinse it off and let it dry.

While he waited, he put some blood from the first tube onto a special glass slide with grids etched on its surface. He selected a low-power lens, placed the slide under the microscope, pressed his face against the eyepieces, and adjusted the focus.

The red blood cells were tiny, and the grid marks helped him to count them. When he had a number he did a quick calculation to determine that the girl had 3.5 million oxygen-carrying red blood cells per cubic millimeter of blood. That was 1 million short of normal—probably a result of the vaginal bleeding.

He rinsed off the gridded slide and dropped another preparation of blood on it. This blood he diluted with hydrochloric acid, to make the red cells disintegrate. That way he could more easily count the white, immune-system cells.

The microscope focused down and he began counting the distinctive white cells. They had lumpy nuclei, surrounded by a thin membrane of clear protoplasm, and in some way that was still anything but clear they were important in fighting infection. When he was finished counting the white cells and making his calculations, he wrote "7,500" on the report form. Normal. That eliminated the possibility that the girl had an infection. . . . If her immune system had been mobilized to fight off an infection, the number would have been far higher.

He made several other observations, noting each one on the form, and then he reached for the slide he had set aside to dry. He placed it on the microscope and swung the high-power lens into place.

The stain made the red cells stand out clearly, and under the high-power lens they looked like tiny round lozenges, thick along the circumference and thin in the center. The white cells seemed normal, too. He made a note and looked at the sheet.

What next?

Platelets.

He needed to examine the platelets or, as they were technically known, thrombocytes. They were tiny things, only visible, really, under the high-power lens, but they were essential to the clotting process.

Scientists hadn't yet worked out all the complex chemistry of clotting, but it was known that injured tissue secreted a protein that made the platelets turn sticky. Being sticky they clumped together, and that formed a plug in the damaged vessel. At the same time the platelets themselves secreted a chemical that triggered a chain reaction among a variety of blood proteins.

It was a complicated, Rube Goldberg process. The blood was full of proteins, and once the platelets had begun the process a chain reaction occurred. One protein activated another, and that activated still another, until, in seconds, molecules of prothrombin began to join end to end, forming hairlike strands. The strands appeared in the blood and instantly tangled, trapping red and white cells, jamming against the plug of platelets, and forming a clot.

Platelet counts were notably difficult to perform, but Bill was, if not good at it, at least competent. He put his eyes back to the microscope, searching for the tiny orange bubbles of protoplasm. He saw none.

Impatiently, he moved the slide a bit and another group of red cells swam into view, but a moment's inspection revealed that there were no little platelets accompanying them. Puzzled now, Bill moved the slide again. And then again. No platelets. Not a one.

Bill raised his face from the microscope. Was he doing something wrong? He *thought* he had done everything properly, but he had never seen blood without platelets before.

If any of the necessary protein factors was missing from a patient's blood, as was the case in hemophilia, the clotting process couldn't be completed. If there were no platelets, it couldn't even begin.

Bill's mind raced, trying to remember if there was a disease that caused platelets to disappear. His lessons jumbled through his mind, but they contained nothing that would explain blood without platelets.

Bill looked at the slides again, with the same result. Explanation or no explanation, the platelets weren't there.

That meant Peggy's denials had been truthful. There was no loss of virginity, no pregnancy, no illegal abortion. She bled because her blood couldn't clot.

But the good news was bad news. If her blood was so

unable to clot that she was bleeding through the walls of her uterus, then she could probably bleed through the membranes of her brain as well. Her reputation had been preserved, but her life might not be. Without platelets, Peggy would surely die.

Bill picked up the telephone and called the Ob-Gyn resident. The man listened to the blood report and then, for a moment, was silent. Bill could tell the resident was puzzled, too, but the man quickly filled the vacuum of knowledge with a label. If there were no thrombocytes, then the girl had . . . well, thrombocytopenia. "Idiopathic" was another good, long word for filling in around an awkward ignorance. It meant unknown. The girl had idiopathic thrombocytopenia.

Bill replaced the telephone receiver in its cradle. He didn't have any idea what that meant, but assumed that the resident would make it his business to find out.

In the meantime . . . Bill remembered the girl's shocked face, her denials, her father's gentle disbelief, her mother's shocked stare. Folding the blood work-up sheet and putting it into the pocket of his white jacket, Bill headed directly for the charity ward to tell her the news and to apologize for the thoughtless preliminary diagnosis.

Bill could tell by the expression of vindication on her face that Peggy understood immediately what he was saying, but for the benefit of her parents he explained it a second time, carefully. Slowly, the mother's hand reached for Peggy's. Her father beamed at her.

Fortunately, the Ob-Gyn resident and the surgical resident entered the curtained-off area before the parents could form the next question: If it wasn't an abortion, then what was it?

In the few minutes since Bill had reported the lack of platelets, the Ob-Gyn man had obviously looked up the condition. Now he talked with authority of "idiopathic thrombocytopenic purpura." Platelets were tiny cells that circulated in the bloodstream and caused clotting, he explained, but in Peggy's case, the spleen was killing them. ITP was serious if untreated . . . but fortunately the treatment was simple. You had a surgeon remove the spleen.

The surgical resident, who had remained silent until now, said that the surgery should be done right away. If she lost more blood, an operation could be dangerous. . . . But no, he said, in response to the father's question, it wasn't a particularly dangerous operation. There was always a risk, of course, but removing the spleen was really rather routine.

Bill watched the girl's face. She didn't ask many questions.

The depth of a patient's natural trust in the medical profession was a source of endless fascination for Bill. The resident had jumped to a conclusion and accused her of willful immorality, and now he was back with a second explanation. Peggy and her family accepted it as truth and signed the surgical permission form without reading it. Outwardly impassive, Bill gave a mental shrug. At least, he told himself, the matter of the abortion had been cleared up.

And anyway, as pretty as the girl was, Bill had other work to do. The old man with the blockage hadn't succeeded in squeezing urine past his swollen prostate for several hours now, and Bill might as well go ahead and lay out the catheterization equipment. He would, he felt certain, be allowed to do the procedure himself. And then there was the elderly woman he had admitted earlier in the evening. Her skin was yellow with jaundice, but she wasn't in pain. That meant the poor lady probably had cancer of the pancreas. He should check on her. For a medical student in a suburban hospital in time of war, there was always something to do. That night, before going to sleep, he finally had the time to review for the upcoming quiz.

The next morning he rose before dawn, groggily dressed himself, assembled his books and notebooks, stuck the stethoscope in his pocket, and followed the wonderful aroma of coffee downstairs to the cafeteria. Breakfast consisted of rubbery scrambled eggs, reconstituted orange juice, and cold toast. It was a measure of his hunger that it appeared appetizing.

As he looked for a clear table that would allow him to open a textbook in front of him while he ate, he spied the surgical resident. The man was bending, exhausted, over a cup of black coffee. Bill paused beside him to inquire how the splenectomy had gone.

The resident looked up at the medical student, his eyes tired. "Oh," he said, "she died."

Bill was stunned.

"Died?" he asked. "From a splenectomy? What happened?"

"I don't know," the resident answered miserably. "I had her sutured up, and she died on the table. Just like that." He turned back to his coffee.

Able to think of nothing else to say, Bill moved on, found a chair, and collapsed into it. The book remained closed. He toyed with his eggs, but his hunger had vanished. The girl's face appeared in his mind, shy, helpless, trusting, denying, frightened . . .

He pushed the tray back, stood, picked up his books, and left the cafeteria. He took the stairs two at a time, into the subbasement, past the NO UNAUTHORIZED PERSONNEL signs, through the double doors, into the autopsy room.

The girl's corpse lay on its back, a block under the base of the skull, head thrown back, half-closed eyes directed at the ceiling. The body cavity was open from throat to pubic bone and the pathologist was directing his assistant's attention to the upper abdomen.

Bill put down his books, pushed up next to the stone slab, and craned his neck to see.

The spleen is normally attached to the rest of the body by a thin pedicle that encloses a large artery and a vein. When the spleen is removed, a ligature is bound tightly around the stump of the pedicle to keep the patient from bleeding to death.

Bill stared beyond the end of the pathologist's pointing finger. The ligature lay free near the stump. It had come off and Peggy had bled to death.

"Who," the pathologist wanted to know, anger in his voice, "who was the surgeon?"

Bill stepped back, his eyes pulled to the Irish face, fair even in death. It took an exercise of will to turn away, but he was late. He picked up his books, pushed his way through the double doors, and rushed to catch his streetcar.

Until that day, the science of hematology had meant little to Bill Harrington. He had studied what had been assigned on the subject, of course, because he was a good student, so he was familiar with the various beasts that live in what is called the bloodstream.

Thanks to the emphasis placed on the subject by his professors, he was particularly familiar with the life cycle of the oxygen-carrying red blood cells. They are born of mother cells, or stem cells as they are called, in the bone marrow, and they pass through a complex series of changes before finally losing their nuclei and turning into the red, thin-centered lozenges that shuttle oxygen to the tissues and carbon dioxide to the lungs.

The life of the red blood cell is a strenuous one. Every few minutes it runs its busy route, squeezing through the capillaries of the lungs and taking on oxygen, swirling through the whirlpools and rapids of the pumping heart, pushing through the capillaries of the tissue, releasing oxygen, and taking on carbon dioxide wastes to carry to the lungs. Every inch of the way it is threatened by bacteria and viruses. The red blood cell is built to last only about three months.

It cannot be allowed to die a natural death, however. For one thing, as carrion it would feed viruses and bacteria and, even more important, the precious iron atoms in its oxygen-carrying hemoglobin molecules might be lost. So the clever forces of evolution arranged for the bloodstream to be populated also by fierce carnivores, amoebalike creatures called phagocytes. The phagocytes are found around the entire bloodstream, attached to the vessel walls and feasting on aging blood cells, but most of them lurk in the liver and spleen.

While they satisfy their voracious appetites, the phagocytes serve a higher function as well. The excrement that the phagocyte pours into the bloodstream is rich in iron, packaged in such a way as to be ready for recycling by the bone-marrow mother cells. And so it is all perfectly balanced, very much like an ecology.

Bill Harrington could and did pass quizzes on the red blood cell, but the other denizens of the bloodstream were more obscure. He knew that the tiny platelet is made in the bone marrow and that it, too, eventually falls prey to the phagocytes. But beyond that, and the fact that it is needed for clotting, Bill could remember little about them. He knew even less about the other cells, the white ones, the immune cells, which live and die with the red cells and platelets in the endlessly swirling river of blood.

It wasn't a subject that Bill was used to thinking about but, this morning, sitting in the streetcar, furious at the incompetent surgeon, abject in his aching pity for the pretty girl, gone now, destroyed by incompetence . . . he struggled to control his rage. What could he do? He wasn't even a doctor yet.

Suddenly, this morning, the subject of platelets was of burning importance. *Idiopathic thrombocytopenic purpura*, the resident had said. It was a mouthful.

The Ob-Gyn resident had said that the phagocytes were killing the platelets before their time. If you removed the spleen, he had added, you removed enough phagocytes so that the platelets would return to normal levels. Then the blood would clot again.

Well, maybe.

In his present frame of mind, Bill wasn't inclined to believe anything either of those two residents had said.

The streetcar clattered to a stop and Bill rose, clutching his books. ITP was apparently an obscure disease, but it ought to be in Cecil's *Textbook of Medicine*. If not, it would certainly be in Wintrobe's *Hematology*.

It was easy to brush up on platelets. Like the red blood cells, they arise from a stem cell deep in the bone marrow. But the platelet, in contrast to the red cell's complex development, comes into being as a bump on the mother cell's surface that enlarges, forms a thin-necked polyp, pinches off, and moves away in the flow of blood. There isn't much to a platelet, and it normally drifts freely in the blood, doing nothing. It normally lives about ten days before being gobbled up by phagocytes.

Idiopathic thrombocytopenic purpura was a little more difficult to find. Later that day, Bill quietly separated himself from his classmates and went to the library. He took down several thick books, carried them to a long mahogany table, and sat down.

Idiopathic thrombocytopenic purpura.

The very first word, "idiopathic," meant unknown. The second indicated that the platelets, or thrombocytes, were few in number. The third word, "purpura," was for the little purple spots. . . .

Spots? He had seen no spots on the girl's skin!

There were usually spots on the skin and on the mucus

membranes of the mouth and throat, the book said. They
looked like measles spots, and were caused by tiny hemorrhages in the skin. Sometimes the spleen was enlarged but
on other occasions it was not. If it had been, Bill would
have detected the swelling when he examined the girl's
midsection.

He read on. Sometimes there was blood in the urine
and stools and sometimes, in women, it was from the vagina. If the patient went untreated he or she might bleed
into the brain and die, but if the spleen was removed the
platelet count rose again and the problem stopped.

Usually, that is. Sometimes, when the spleen was removed, the condition got worse.

As the resident had explained, one theory held that the
phagocytes in the spleen were killing all the platelets. But
other researchers observed that while normal capillaries
clamped down when cut, helping to stop the bleeding, the
capillaries of ITP victims did not. Therefore, they reasoned, ITP must involve the secretion of some damaging
chemical that paralyzed the capillaries and, at the same
time, somehow damaged the platelet's mother cells in the
bone marrow. As near as Bill could tell, one theory was as
good as the other.

He wasn't surprised to discover that ITP was a lot more
mysterious than the resident had let on, but at the same
time he wasn't prepared for the incredible complexity he
found. The blood flowed thick with complex molecules,
all interacting with one another, and what one scientific
paper established the next seemed to disprove. For every
rule there seemed to be an exception. Every elusive fact,
when finally grasped, popped like a balloon and left only
questions.

Finally, reluctantly, Bill closed the books and replaced
them on the shelf. He first had to become a real doctor,
and there was a quiz tomorrow. There was always a quiz
tomorrow, and another one the day after that.

The year 1945 passed, one quiz after another, and young Bill Harrington kept up the effort that would one day win him scholastic honors. He studied kidneys and the retina of the eye. He memorized the names of bacteria and learned to set bones. He delivered babies, inoculated guinea pigs, and learned to use the wonderful new antibiotics. One patient's face blended into another, men and women almost indistinguishable in his fact-crammed memory. But he never forgot the pretty, frightened face of the Irish girl on the ward, and how it had become a relaxed dead face on the autopsy block. And his driving interest in hematology grew and grew until it became his future.

As the doctors came back from the war, Bill attached himself to one of the hematologists, Dr. William C. Moloney, and his informal apprenticeship began. During his internship and a two-year residency at Boston City Hospital, he spent every spare minute studying the relationships among the enigmatic creatures populating the human bloodstream.

As he learned more and more about the creatures he became increasingly fascinated as well by the nature of the river of serum in which they traveled. Through the microscope the serum looked to him like ordinary water, and mostly it was. But it contained some extraordinary molecules that were far too small to be visualized under the highest power. One set of those molecules were called antibodies, and they allowed the body to perform awesome tricks of self-defense.

Long before it was known that life was based on Tinkertoy molecules, back when the heavens were composed of a blue crystal dome upon which angels danced, back when the world consisted of earth, air, fire, and water, curious men and women had seen the magic of the antibodies and noted it.

It was curious, the Chinese said. If you took the scabs

from a smallpox victim, and if you ground up those scabs, and then inhaled them . . . why, if you did all that, you wouldn't get smallpox at all. In the Middle East, such powders were rubbed into cuts made in the skin of young girls. Girls, who weren't much prized under any circumstances, were completely worthless if their faces were pitted by smallpox.

By the time hematology became the object of Bill Harrington's aspirations, it was known that the antibodies were somehow responsible for such immune reactions. They were special molecules that could identify and latch onto the proteins on the surface of bacteria. In fact, they could glom onto virtually any alien protein molecule.

That ability was no longer, in Bill Harrington's time, totally magic. Proteins, after all, were recognized as big molecules of varying sizes, shapes, and electrical charges. It would be relatively easy, if you were Mother Nature, to make an antiprotein molecule.

An antiprotein molecule would be able to recognize its victim by Braille, so to speak, and latch onto it. There would be many kinds of antibodies, and each would be programmed for a specific protein—a protein, say, from the eye of a newt. By that theory, there would have to be thousands, millions, billions of different kinds of antibodies. It was enough to boggle a medical student's mind but, for Mother Nature, a type of molecule with a billion variations was not unreasonable.

Whatever their shapes, sizes, and methods of operation, antibodies had dramatic effects. You couldn't see the antibodies to identify them, but you could tell they were there by their actions. If you introduced bacteria into a petri dish of serum containing antibodies against that particular breed of bacteria, for instance, the antibodies would immediately form a gooey gel around each creature. As the bacteria swam frantically, bumping into one another, they stuck solidly and helplessly together. Were they in the body, they would form an irresistible morsel for a hungry phagocyte.

As Bill completed his residency in Boston, the new knowledge about antibodies was revolutionizing medicine. All over the world, young would-be hematologists were sticking one another's fingers for drops of blood.

They were learning that, as some people are Capricorns and others are Tauruses, some are type O and some are AB. Tests could be performed to find out whose blood proteins matched with whose, and sick people were being transfused with blood so closely matched with their own that their immune systems didn't recognize it as foreign. Allergies were beginning to be understood, dimly, as involving the immune system. New tests were being devised and new immunization techniques tested.

But the realization was dawning that the body's ability to send out antibodies after specific invaders, while impressive, wasn't nearly so magical as its ability to recognize those invaders in the first place. How did it distinguish between its own proteins and those of a bacterium? Or even those of another human?

Yet, somehow, it made the distinction. Otherwise, it might accidentally attack its own brain cells, or its own kidney cells, or its own . . .

. . . platelets?

The question was not a total shot in the dark. During World War II soldiers took quinine tablets to prevent malaria. The quinine ended up in the blood cells and changed them enough to prevent the malarial parasites from taking hold. Despite the soldiers' universal dislike for the taste of quinine, it worked very well.

Or at least, Bill discovered in the course of his reading, it usually worked well. But sometimes the soldier developed a strange anemia in which his antibodies attacked and killed his own red blood cells.

The theory was that the quinine, as it slipped into the

blood cell protein, changed its shape slightly. Suddenly, the protein seemed somehow different and, in the Braille of the immune system, it was mistaken for something alien and became a target for attack.

In Bill Harrington's mind there was another suggestive piece of evidence regarding ITP. Sometimes when a woman had ITP and became pregnant, the baby was born with ITP as well. But the baby, with time, got better. It was almost as though some damaging substance had passed through the placenta and into the child and then, after birth, was eventually destroyed.

In the meantime Bill, driven by his ambition to understand ITP, was adapting well to the life of a hematologist. His hands had a slight tremor, but through concentration he mastered one of the most difficult feats of dexterity in the hematology laboratory—inserting a tiny needle into a vein in the tail of a newborn mouse. His colleagues said that if you had to have someone plunge a needle into you, then you wanted that someone to be Dr. Harrington. Bill, for his part, liked the people, liked the patients, liked the work. He didn't even mind sticking his own finger.

In hematology, someone's finger is always getting pricked. It is difficult to ask the fellow at the next bench for a spot of his blood when you know his finger is as abused as your own. If you ask, he will probably offer to stick your finger for you if you can't bear to do it yourself. So it is easier, everything else being equal, to stick your own finger. You don't have to like it, you just have to do it—and, in the name of curiosity and career, Bill Harrington was willing to do a lot of distasteful things. He worked hard and it paid off.

In 1950, his residency finally completed, he landed a fellowship in hematology under Dr. Carl V. Moore at the prestigious Barnes Hospital in St. Louis. By the time he arrived in July, his suspicion about ITP had grown into what passes, in a scientist, for conviction.

July is a month of confusion in the medical world. Medical students become interns in unfamiliar hospitals. Interns become residents and are assigned strange new duties. Instructors leave to become assistant professors and are replaced by young men and women who, just a week or so before, were fellows. The result is pandemonium. Bill had little time, in July, to remember the frightened Irish eyes.

The pressure of July is conducive, as well, to the formation of new alliances. Barnes officials had arranged for Bill and the other new fellows to room together in a large house during their first summer in St. Louis, and the result was several strong friendships.

Bill Harrington very naturally developed a comradeship with a young man from North Carolina, Dr. James William Hollingsworth, more frequently addressed simply as Holly. Bill and Holly ate lunch together, argued a little politics, and made jokes about the Civil War. When there was time for woolgathering, they shared their dreams.

Holly was studying the immune system and had been passing serum back and forth between rabbits, guinea pigs, and other animals, so he was easily intrigued by Bill's idea about the body's being immune to its own platelets. As the two young doctors kicked the idea around, the rough outlines of an experiment developed.

The question was simple. What would happen if they took a pint of blood from an ITP patient and gave it to a normal subject? Say, for the sake of argument, they gave it to Bill. . . .

If ITP was caused by the spleen, nothing would happen. But if it was caused by some antibodies circulating in the serum, then those antibodies should attack Bill's platelets and they should dwindle in number. He should get a sort of, well, pseudo-ITP.

Or maybe something different would happen, or maybe . . . who knew?

It was probably as complicated as everything else in biology seemed to be, of course, and an experiment like that probably wouldn't work. They usually didn't.

Still.

Wouldn't it be elegant if it *did* work?

The trick would be in detecting and recording the effect, since a single pint of ITP blood probably wouldn't make all that much difference to the person who received it.

As Bill and Holly talked about it, they realized the problems were many. In the first place, since it was hospital policy to remove the spleens of ITP patients immediately, and since those ITP patients usually improved dramatically as a result, it would be very difficult to find an active case to donate the necessary blood.

They also needed a matching blood type, since a mismatch would cause a reaction that would obscure the ITP effect, whatever it was. Bill was type O and Holly was type B.

If the opportunity ever presented itself, they promised one another, they would try it. The one with the matching blood would be the guinea pig.

August was almost as hectic as July had been, as Harrington worked to integrate himself into Dr. Moore's research on iron metabolism. Then, one Sunday in early September, one of the most seriously ill ITP patients that Bill had ever seen was admitted to the hospital. He recognized his opportunity and immediately ran to fetch Holly.

As the two hematology fellows examined the middle-aged woman and leafed through her thick record from previous admissions, they became increasingly excited. She had had her spleen removed a few months earlier and, obviously, that hadn't helped much. Her blood smear on admission had shown virtually no platelets, her skin was covered with tiny hemorrhagic spots, and her black stools indicated that blood was seeping through the walls of her intestines. It was a terrible case and that, for Bill and Holly, was wonderful.

She also had type O blood, which meant Bill would be the recipient. In their enthusiasm they explained to her what they were about to do and why, and she immediately became a co-conspirator.

If the experiment was to stand up to scientific scrutiny, Bill and Holly knew, they would need plenty of documentation. The woman's history was thoroughly recorded in her thick medical record, but they would need data on Bill as well. They would need blood smears to document the level of his platelets before the experiment, and other smears later to prove the level had fallen . . . assuming it had. Bill also insisted on bone marrow smears, in case the patient's ITP antibodies acted against the platelets' mother cells, instead of the platelets themselves. Bill could stick his own finger, but Holly would have to do the marrow tap. They went to the lab.

Sunday afternoons are quiet even at a big teaching hospital like Barnes, and the laboratory was empty. Bill washed his finger with alcohol and stabbed the lancet into it. The blood went on the slide and under the microscope. Bill and Holly could tell at a glance that the count was roughly normal, and they set the slides aside for later. Then Bill lay down on a table while Holly readied the instruments for the marrow tap.

Holly would have been perfectly willing to play the guinea pig himself. He would have done it without a thought, in fact. He would have taken the woman's blood with hardly a thought, but . . . but a marrow tap . . . yeesh.

Holly had done enough bone marrow aspirations on other people to know that they hurt. Suddenly he was glad the woman's blood type had been O and not B. As he bathed the center of Bill's breastbone with iodine and then washed off the iodine with alcohol, he admired his friend's stoic demeanor.

Bill's expression didn't change as Holly inserted the novocaine-containing needle beneath the skin on the center of Bill's chest. As the needle darted back and forth and the skin puffed up with painkilling liquid, the Irishman's expression still didn't change. He didn't wince either when the needle pierced the sensitive membrane that covered the bone, and squirted a drop of novocaine beneath it.

Holly laid aside the novocaine syringe and picked up a large stainless-steel instrument that looked like a miniature auger. The business end was like an ice pick, but it had large crossbar handles.

Bill stared up at the ceiling as Holly pressed the point against the bone, directly over his heart, and pushed. As he pressed, Holly twisted the instrument back and forth, working it into the bone. There was no pain yet, since the bone's membrane had been deadened, but Holly knew from watching his patients that nothing could deaden the awful feeling that someone was driving a stake into your heart. Yet Bill didn't flinch.

When he was satisfied with the depth of the ice pick in the bone, Holly stopped pushing and, holding the instrument in place, withdrew a long, thin wire from its top. That opened a channel down the center of the ice pick, converting it into a hypodermic needle. Holly fastened a syringe barrel to the top of the instrument, grabbed its plunger, and withdrew it sharply. Bill's eyes widened and his body twitched almost imperceptibly.

A tiny quantity of a watery, maroon substance gushed into the syringe and was quickly transferred to a slide, for the record.

The next steps were obvious and routine. A pint of blood was drawn both from the patient and from Bill, and Bill's was given to the patient. Who knew—it might do her some good.

Then, back in the laboratory, the ITP blood was set to drip into Bill's veins. While the transfusion took place, Bill settled in with a medical journal while Holly sterilized his equipment in preparation for a second, posttransfusion bone marrow aspiration.

As soon as the transfusion was complete, a process that took about ten minutes, Holly stuck Bill's finger a second time and did a platelet count. The result was surprising, and both men took turns looking through the microscope. Already there was a modest, but very real, diminution of platelets.

Then Bill lay back on the table and stared at the ceiling while Holly again slid the novocaine needle into the skin of his chest, about an inch from where the first marrow sample had been taken.

After the second bone marrow sample was drawn, Bill slowly sat up on the table and put his shirt back on. He felt . . . not right. He didn't say anything to Holly, because he didn't feel sick in any specific way, just . . . uneasy.

He slipped off the table and helped Holly clean things up, and then they went to dinner. Holly occasionally glanced at his friend, thinking he looked a little . . . a little . . . a little something. A little peaked. Maybe, Holly thought, the bone marrow exams were getting to him.

As they ate, Holly suggested to Bill that no more marrows needed to be done, but Bill dismissed the idea. Everything was going so well and he wasn't about to jeopardize the experiment with a cowardly decision. Besides, he assured Holly, he felt fine. Which, he told himself, he did. More or less.

After dinner, another drop of blood from Bill's finger indicated that the platelets were still decreasing. For the first time, the young scientists allowed themselves to think that they might be in the midst of a really important discovery. Whatever the ITP factor was, it was potent stuff!

Bill lay down on the laboratory table for the third marrow tap and Holly stepped to the lab bench to prepare the instruments. As he worked he glanced back at Bill, who was lying with his head toward the bench, so that his face was out of view. Holly stopped working.

Something had attracted his attention. Had Bill twitched?

Holly looked harder. Because of the angle, the only skin Holly could see was the tops of Bill's ears.

"Bill . . . ?" the southerner asked uneasily. "Bill?"

This time it was unmistakable. Bill twitched.

Instantly, Holly relaxed. The twitch was such a dramatic one . . . he knew immediately that it was a joke. Bill had a strange sense of humor.

"C'mon, Yankee boy," Holly said. "We've got work to do. . . ." And then he stopped, staring at the tops of Bill's ears. They had begun to turn blue.

Instantly Holly was beside the table, but the convulsion, or whatever it was, was over. Maybe it wasn't a convulsion; maybe it was just fainting, from the marrow taps. That made sense to Holly.

Perhaps, he suggested again, they should cut out the bone marrow taps. Enough was enough. But Bill rejected the suggestion instantly; fainting or no fainting, he wasn't about to mar what was otherwise shaping up to be a perfect experiment. Reluctantly, Holly went on with the preparations.

Again and again they pricked Bill's finger and counted his platelets, and each time the count was a little lower than it had been before. By late evening little hemorrhagic spots appeared around Bill's ankles.

By midnight and the fourth bone marrow tap, Bill had all the classic signs: If he had walked into the emergency room as a patient he would have been immediately diagnosed as having ITP, and emergency surgery would have been scheduled to remove his spleen. There was no doubt in either man's mind that the experiment was conclusive. All that needed to be done now was to wait for the effects to wear off.

As they walked home through the muggy St. Louis night, Bill was quietly jubilant. The experiment had succeeded beyond his wildest imagination.

At 8 A.M. the next morning Bill and Holly were back at the hospital, joining Dr. Moore's group for rounds. They followed him from bed to bed, examining leukemia patients, anemia patients, and finally the woman with ITP. The case was notable, Dr. Moore explained, because the removal of the spleen hadn't helped.

Bill, not yet ready to explain his self-experiment, tried to look only moderately interested. But as the group moved away from the bed, a student asked Dr. Moore what usually happened in ITP when removal of the spleen didn't help.

"Well," the professor said, keeping his somber voice low enough so that the woman couldn't hear, "they usually die."

The words touched some vital part of Bill's psyche. His diaphragm convulsed involuntarily and he emitted a laughing noise so loud that Dr. Moore looked up sharply, obviously shocked and angered at what appeared to be his new fellow's insensitivity.

Bill reddened under the stare, searching for words, stammering out the story.

As Dr. Moore listened the expression on his face slowly changed from anger to mere irritation, from irritation to comprehension, and from comprehension to relief.

Over a long career as a scientist-teacher, Dr. Moore had had many residents and fellows who took themselves, and their work, too seriously. In their enthusiasm they jumped to conclusions, misread experiments, and . . . and very few of them could even do a decent platelet count. He automatically assumed Bill and Holly had merely seen what they wanted to see in the slides. Bill's platelet count was probably perfectly normal.

A laboratory technician had been making rounds with the group, and Dr. Moore ordered her to take Dr. Harrington back to the laboratory and do a platelet count. Certain the technician's count would show Bill's blood to be normal, Dr. Moore headed for his office to catch up on paperwork. The rest of the group, fascinated, followed Bill and the technician.

A few minutes later the technician was in Dr. Moore's office. Not only did Bill have no platelets, she reported, he had characteristic hemorrhages under the skin around the ankles.

Frowning, Dr. Moore pushed the paperwork aside and rose from his desk. He wanted to see the slides himself. A few minutes later he lifted his face from the microscope and agreed with the technician. His eyes rested on Bill, who was standing aside nervously. Seeing the expression on his chief's face, Bill was, for the first time, somewhat apprehensive.

He answered Dr. Moore's questions as fully as he knew how and, when the orders were given, meekly followed the nurse to the clinical area. She led him to a private room and gave him a split-up-the-back hospital gown.

The private room, Dr. Moore made clear to all concerned, was chosen so that Bill wouldn't be subjected to constant inquiry by his peers. Dr. Moore had no idea what the ultimate consequences of the experiment would be, but he knew he wanted his patient kept quiet, in hopes of preventing any major internal bleeding. Holly was allowed to visit his friend briefly, but most of the fellows and medical students had to content themselves with an occasional peak through the door.

While news of his deeds quickly dominated the hospital rumor mill, Bill himself sat, bored, in the eye of the hurricane, reading medical journals and trying not to think of the "what ifs."

The first what if, of course, was what if his platelets didn't come back? He had blithely assumed they would . . . but then, he had also assumed that he wouldn't get much of an effect from a single pint of ITP blood.

And if his platelets didn't come back, would removing his spleen help? A splenectomy hadn't helped the woman whose blood he had taken.

And what if, and what if, and what if he bled into his brain?

He would be a cripple.

The important thing was not to lie down. The hemorrhages under his skin were confined to his lower legs, so far, and, while blood had begun to seep into his stools and urine, the internal bleeding seemed mostly confined to the lower part of his body. Perhaps if he didn't lie down, if he remained sitting up, he could keep from bleeding into his brain.

Or maybe if he bled into his brain he wouldn't be a cripple at all.

Maybe he would die.

And what then?

Suddenly, Bill's church seemed very important to him. He placed a call to a priest and explained what he had done. What was the church's attitude toward self-experimentation?

Several medical scientists at Barnes had dropped what they were doing to focus on Bill's case, and to try to puzzle out what was happening. They came around to sit by his bed and ask him questions. Bill tried to be as helpful as he could, though, as a scientist himself, he knew the researchers would be of little immediate help.

Time after time he let the hematology technician stick his finger, and time after time the readings were the same. He had no platelets. Zero.

That night, sitting up in bed, propped up by a mountain of pillows, he dozed fitfully. He hadn't realized how difficult it was to sleep sitting up.

By the next day Bill's platelet counts were still running at zero but, with the passage of time and scientific thought, Dr. Moore's apprehension had begun to subside somewhat. ITP was apparently caused by some circulating factor in the patient's blood, just as Bill had reasoned, and that factor was probably an antibody against a protein in the platelets. As soon as the ITP antibodies were exhausted, the scientists predicted, Bill's platelets would reappear.

The scientists were more than optimistic—they were excited. There had been theories that the body might, under certain circumstances, become immune to itself and attack its own cells. There was, for instance, the idea that malaria drugs could lead to such a phenomenon . . . but the picture was rather fuzzy. Bill Harrington's self-experiment was the clearest demonstration to date that there was a certain category of diseases that were "autoimmune."

Dr. Moore didn't fully share their excitement until five days later, when the first platelets reappeared in his student's blood. Eyes reddened by five consecutive sleepless nights, an ecstatic Bill Harrington began accepting the congratulations of a steady stream of visitors.

In the weeks following any major discovery, the laboratory involved becomes a madhouse. At Barnes in St. Louis, the remainder of the summer and the autumn of 1950 were consumed by dozens of experiments. Medical students, scientists, secretaries, laboratory workers—even Dr. Moore himself—allowed small, measured amounts of ITP blood to be injected into their veins. They received no more than a small fraction of what Bill Harrington had taken. Later others were given larger amounts but under carefully controlled conditions.

As the winter passed in frenzied effort, the experiments demonstrated that the ITP antibodies were indeed very powerful, and very effective at destroying platelets. The results set the mind to wondering . . . how many other diseases were autoimmune?

By spring the discoveries in St. Louis were the talk of the medical world. On April 30 Bill read his paper before a rapt audience at the forty-third annual meeting of the American Society for Clinical Investigation. Afterward, the bars were filled with scientists who wondered, and theorized, and dreamed of finding other diseases that could be laid to an autoimmune reaction.

And so it was that a disastrous experience with a frightened young patient changed the life of a medical student, and he in turn changed the history of medicine.

In the three decades that have passed since Bill Harrington poisoned himself with an ITP patient's blood, several other mysterious diseases have been found to be due to autoimmunity. In lupus, for instance, the patient—usually a young woman—makes antibodies that destroy her kidneys and change the shape of her body. In myasthenia gravis, the patient is progressively weakened by an antibody that attacks the specialized terminals that attach nerves to muscles. Many scientists now believe that rheumatoid arthritis is an autoimmune disease as well.

Both Dr. William Harrington and Dr. James William Hollingsworth went on to become successful in medicine. Dr. Hollingsworth is chief of medicine at the Veterans Administration Hospital in San Diego, and is no longer known as Holly. *His* students, he emphasizes, would never try such an experiment: Bill's brush with death frightened Dr. Hollingsworth so thoroughly that he actively counsels his doctors against thoughtless self-experimentation of any sort, no matter how minor.

Dr. Harrington, now recognized as the world's leading expert on ITP, lives on the opposite coast, where he serves as Distinguished Professor of Medicine at the University of Miami Medical School.

When asked about his youthful experiment, as he frequently is, Dr. Harrington settles back for a long story. It all started, he says, in Boston.

It was wartime then, and a medical student had a lot of clout, and he was doing admitting work. One night a young girl came to the ward, a remarkably beautiful girl. She was bleeding from the vagina and an idiot of a resident told her she had had an abortion . . . a charge that she tearfully denied.

It would never happen now, of course.

ITP, as the humblest medical student must know, is an autoimmune disease characterized by the death of platelets and unexplained bleeding. Even today there is no cure, but thanks to the later work of Harrington and others, its effects can be mitigated by the use of a variety of drug therapies, including steroids and the anticancer compound vincristine.

And, thanks to Bill Harrington, it is almost always diagnosed correctly and early. No modern resident would mistake it for postabortion hemorrhage.

THE FASTEST MAN
ON EARTH

December, 1954.

The ugly blue-gray overcast stretched all the way from the Sacramento Mountains in the east to the San Andres range on the opposite horizon. The clouds had remained unbroken since dawn.

Dr. John Paul Stapp stood, in his flight suit, on the desert floor, just a few miles from where the atomic age had been born in wind and fire. He stared at the bright spot in the clouds that hung halfway between the peaks of the Sacramentos and the zenith.

Occasionally the brightness wavered as the boiling clouds moved across it. That meant, he knew, that parts of the overcast were thin. That meant that there might be a break.

Five minutes of sunshine. That was all he needed, five minutes.

Dr. Stapp looked around him. Even with the muted sun, there was almost enough light. There was enough, for instance, for the red and white rocket sled to cast a fuzzy shadow. The two small hills to the south, toward Mexico, had swelled to the size of a mountain, so there was enough light for a mirage. There was more than sufficient light to satisfy the news photographers, who were sitting in and on the parked jeeps.

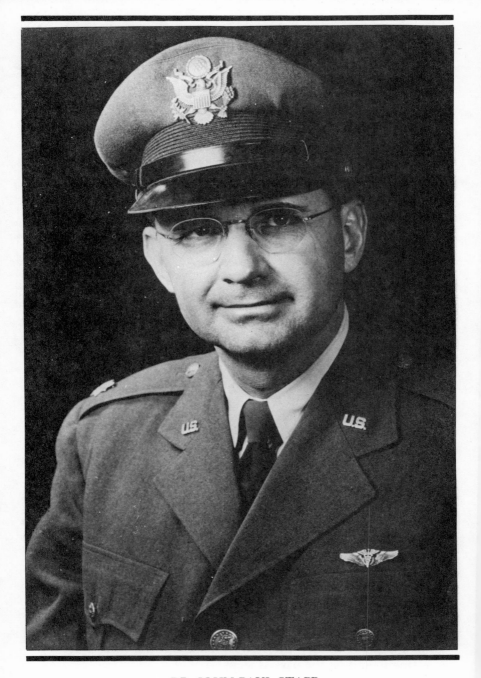

DR. JOHN PAUL STAPP

It was almost bright enough for the high-speed scientific cameras in the sled and chase plane.

Almost, but not quite.

Maybe there would be a break in the cloud cover and they could get on with it.

Sure, there would be a break. That was what he told the crew, anyway. Even in science, you've got to have faith.

"*Testing*," said the blockhouse speaker, booming out over the desert. "*Testing, one, two* . . ."

Perhaps he should go get strapped in and wait for a bright spot. If the sun came out and the restraints weren't fastened, it might cloud over again before they could get ready.

Of all the bad luck. How could you anticipate clouds over White Sands?

There was always sun in the desert, which was one reason he loved it so much. He loved the expanse of valley and the mirage lakes, loved to fly in the brilliant blue sky, loved to lie and be washed by the sun.

It was an environment that was belligerently different from the one he had grown up in, as part of a missionary family, in Brazil. Clouds evoked emotions that sparked memories of delirium and malaria.

Dr. Stapp paced, impatiently, looking frequently at the ugly blue-gray sky. He conferred briefly with his engineer, an enlisted man from Baltimore.

"It'll clear up," Dr. Stapp said.

The news photographers sat like vultures, with the patience of people who are getting paid by the hour. Idly, one of them raised a Speed Graphic and snapped a picture.

Their editors liked the story of the daring Air Force flight surgeon, and were mesmerized by the danger. Dr. Stapp had tried to explain to them that there was no danger but, like the Air Force brass, they refused to listen.

Well, maybe the attention would do the program some good. Maybe it would make his superiors leave him alone and trust him to do his job.

The flight surgeon turned toward the rocket sled. Several more cameras clicked.

A jeep started up and moved onto the dirt road paralleling the steel tracks. It bounced northward, horn honking, a plume of dust rising behind it.

The tracks were set on concrete strips, and there was a deep ditch between them. At the far end of the run, fiberboard dams had been fitted between the tracks, and earlier a tank truck had gone out to the track's end and filled the resulting pools with water.

Once they were filled, the pools had to be carefully watched. The only open water for miles around, they were a magnet for birds, coyotes, and other desert creatures.

If Dr. Stapp hit a Mexican chickadee at four hundred miles an hour . . . that could do a lot of damage to the overbite. Well, the honking jeep should scare them away.

The only permanent solution, Dr. Stapp knew, was to build a separate pond a mile or so away and dedicate it to the coyotes and birds. But that would take money, so he just didn't think about it.

A breeze puffed across the valley, sweeping away the dust cloud left by the jeep. Dr. Stapp hoped the wind would stay down. He didn't need wind—he needed sun.

Five minutes was all he needed. Just five minutes.

He walked toward the sled.

It sat high atop the tracks, an ungraceful apparatus of struts and pipes that the Stapp crew had christened *Sonic Wind Number One*.

The rockets took up most of the space in the rear of the sled, and the seat was in front. Dr. Stapp grabbed a strut, put a foot on the rail, and swung himself up.

Two hundred feet away, cameras clicked.

A junior medical officer, a member of Dr. Stapp's team who had ridden the sled himself and who would serve as flight surgeon for this test, climbed up beside him. The sled mechanic climbed up on the other side. He had ridden the sled as well. But nobody had made a ride like this.

"Strap me in," Dr. Stapp said, settling into the chair. "It'll clear."

Dr. Stapp relaxed, letting them spin the web of straps around his body.

It was, in large part, the straps that made it possible for humans to ride the sled. Every restraint had a specific function with a history, a theory, an animal test behind it.

Earlier scientists had used human corpses to test the upper limits of physical endurance, but Dr. Stapp had started out with anesthetized animals. Monkeys. Bears. Pigs.

Pigs were very good test subjects. They were a lot like men. The animals, and their sometimes gruesome injuries, had helped him design the straps.

Dr. Stapp knew exactly what he was doing, and that, he told the brass again and again, made it perfectly safe.

But what if something went wrong? . . .

The flight surgeon's response would have made perfect sense to another pilot.

Something go wrong?

Why, that's no problem.

You just don't let anything go wrong. You see, that's what makes it so safe.

Dr. Stapp was content with test pilot logic, but other people, who sat behind desks in Washington, weren't.

The editors of the newsmagazines obviously didn't understand, either. If they had, they wouldn't have sent so many photographers.

Let the editors think it was dangerous, then, if that was

what it took. Let the brass think it was stupid. John Stapp
knew better. He wasn't going to waste time agonizing. If
his pulse got a little rapid when he climbed onto the sled,
well, it was a normal physiological reaction. The beating
heart meant fear only if you wanted to interpret it that way.

To a scientist, it was simply data.

The flight surgeon handed Dr. Stapp the crash helmet,
and he slipped it over his head.

With science, the human body could endure awesome
forces without injury. With science, Dr. Stapp could survive the sled, and if his heart beat a little fast it was because the heart knew no science. With scientists going
before them and calculating the forces, pilots could survive
ejection at Mach 2.

With science, military men and civilians alike could survive automobile accidents.

Everyone was afraid of polio, but anybody who had
ever spent any time in an emergency room or a morgue
knew the big killer of children wasn't polio. And it wasn't
cancer that killed the young mother or father, either.

The peculiar plague of the 20th century was getting pul-
verized. If people behind desks wanted to worry, they
ought to worry about the tens of thousands of Americans
who died each year, needlessly, on the highways.

No, what Dr. Stapp was doing wasn't stupid—and it
wasn't trivial, either.

Unfortunately, "studying the forces that mashed people" didn't have the ring of a scientific endeavor. But it
was, and it was a very critical one at that.

Dr. Stapp called his science biodynamics, and if his
heart raced toward the end of the countdown it might
have something to do with scientific excitement. The
equations that came out of the sled runs were leading him
and his fellow scientists to the very frontier between biology and physics.

That was what nobody seemed to understand. It wasn't the thunder of the rockets that made him do what he did, and it wasn't the euphoria he felt when each ride was over. Riding the sled, he told reporters, wasn't habit-forming.

What motivated him was the siren call of the equations, and the knowledge that he was doing something important. And that, he would admit if asked, was habit-forming.

Unfortunately, the reporters rarely asked.

Now an Air Force ambulance rolled to a stop beside the parked jeeps. The driver fumbled with the lid of a paper coffee cup.

Before the crew strapped his helmet to the headrest, Dr. Stapp looked up one last time at the ugly, overcast sky. There were no clearings.

It'll break, he reassured the flight surgeon. Let's just wait until it does, and then we'll be ready and we can go.

Clouds over Alamogordo! Of all the rotten, rotten luck!

Far to the west, a buzzard circled beneath the blue-gray ceiling.

The flight suit was hot. The bright spot in the clouds climbed higher, and the mirage mountains shimmered behind him.

When the mechanic and the flight surgeon were finished, Dr. Stapp was totally immobilized by straps around his ankles, knees, thighs, elbows, wrists, and chest. Without the straps the air blast would pull his limbs out into the windstream and break them. Animal runs had taught him that.

The mechanic had left the chest straps a little loose, to make the waiting easier. Dr. Stapp, his head immobilized, stared straight ahead, eyes focused on the horizon, where distance made the tracks seem to come together.

Slowly, the bright spot in the clouds moved higher and higher. The photographers tinkered with their equipment.

The ambulance driver finished his coffee and began idly tearing the empty cup to shreds.

Dr. Stapp waited.

From the beginning there had been clues that, under the proper set of circumstances, the human body could tolerate unbelievable impacts. There were legends of people who had fallen from airplanes and survived, usually after landing in a snowbank or freshly plowed field. And there was the 16-year-old boy who had plunged 244 feet from the Golden Gate Bridge to the water, and survived. Many such incidents had been documented.

Such improbable, narrow escapes were clearly due, in part, to the fact that the falling people had struck something soft, which absorbed some of the energy. The position of the body at the moment of impact was also critical.

The boy who jumped from the bridge hit the water at 72.8 miles per hour, and at that velocity water isn't a very soft substance. But he landed feet first, a position that allowed him to cut through the water and transmitted the shock more or less equally through his body. He escaped with a broken shoulder and back . . . minor, given the circumstances.

The people who survived high falls onto land, however, usually hit flat on their backs, which also allowed the shock to be averaged throughout the body.

Dr. Stapp's colleagues had collected hundreds of such stories, some better documented than others. They sat in their offices late at night, puzzling over autopsy reports and computing exactly what forces were involved in the mashing process. At meetings they debated for hours, concocting and discarding theories about why one fall victim died while another lived.

One of the first pieces of jargon invented to serve the new science of biodynamics was the "G."

As Dr. Stapp explained to the reporters, the G was a measure of force . . . mass times acceleration, for those

who knew their physics. The kind of force being measured in this instance was the force that, in a rapidly accel-
erating elevator, pushed you down and seemed to increase
your weight.

Unless, of course, the elevator was falling. In that case,
you would feel lighter.

One G represented the normal pull of gravity. If you
got twice that in an elevator, you would wish you were
someplace else. The boy who had jumped off the Golden
Gate Bridge absorbed 35 Gs at the moment of impact.

The G forces could come instantly, Dr. Stapp said, as
happened when a suicide landed on a Park Avenue sidewalk. Or they could be spread over a millisecond or so, in
which case the outcome was often quite different. One
man had tried to end his life by diving from a high window, but survived the fall because he landed on the roof of
a passing car, crushing it. Many of the Gs were expended
in crushing the car top, a process that, while quick, wasn't
instantaneous.

Though supersonic aircraft crashes were a relatively
minor cause of death in the United States, compared to
automobile accidents, it was the Air Force and not the civilian bureaucracy that supported Dr. Stapp and most of
his colleagues.

The service had a historical commitment to the men
who flew its machines. As those machines boomed
through Mach 1 and edged toward Mach 2, the fragile human bodies they carried needed to be increasingly well
protected.

And that meant, Dr. Stapp said, that they needed to
know the limits of human endurance.

It was patently obvious to the flight surgeon that there
was only one direct way of finding out how much force
flesh and bone could stand, and that was by subjecting
flesh and bone to that much force.

There were various ways of doing that, all of them involving either a sudden acceleration or a sudden stop.

Scientists before Dr. Stapp had used a variety of dynamic stress devices. Animals and men rode rigid swings that fell to the bottom of their arc, hit a projection, and came to a jarring stop. One group built a chair that was attached by huge rubber bands to a giant slingshot.

But the best way to pit G forces against flesh and bone, Dr. Stapp thought, was to use a rocket sled that would attain a high speed and then be brought to a very sudden halt.

The Air Force officers wanted the information Dr. Stapp offered to provide, but they were ambivalent about his machinery. What the bright young flight surgeon had in mind looked, well . . . dangerous.

They didn't order him to do it. They didn't even ask him. But neither did they tell him not to.

So Dr. Stapp's work began near Edwards Air Force Base in California, under less than auspicious circumstances. The group's first rocket sled was a small one, and the equipment was mostly procured through what the military calls "midnight requisitions."

Even the present test site, next to the White Sands National Monument in New Mexico, was hand-me-down. The thirty-five-hundred-foot track was designed to fling missiles into the air, and when that program had been completed the facility qualified as a white elephant.

To Dr. Stapp, it was a godsend.

Now, sitting strapped to the sled, he scanned the sky. Nothing.

It was blue-gray, from mountain range to mountain range.

Again, the honking jeep ran the track.

Sonic Wind Number One, like the sled in California, was held to the earth by many feet that curved around the flat bead at the top of the steel track. Wheels weren't necessary. At the speeds involved, the feet would be held away from the rails by vibration, what the engineers called frictional chatter.

One of the most critical parts of the apparatus was the braking mechanism. For the equations to work out, the scientists needed to slow and stop the sled within a specified distance, building up a precalculated G force. The faster the stop, the higher the Gs.

The first sled had relied on mechanical brakes, but that system had its problems. On the forty-eighth human run in California, for instance, the sled's brakes had jammed. From a peak speed of 129.5 miles an hour, the sled had come to a dead stop in just 12 feet.

The man, who had ridden facing backward, had a tender tailbone and a sore back for a few days.

That and the time a man had blacked out several times after a high-speed run were the worst incidents recorded by the human test program. Dr. Stapp wished fervently that his superiors would take more comfort from that fact.

There was his own broken wrist, of course, but that was nothing. He was annoyed when the reporters mentioned it in their stories.

The point was that everything was done first with animals. By the time Dr. Stapp climbed aboard a sled, there were no surprises left.

The animal runs told the scientists what humans could do safely and, just as important, what they shouldn't try.

For instance, early in the program there was the notion that the pilot of a high-speed aircraft might be safer if the ejection seat blew him into the air blast head first. That was, after all, how a high diver hit the water.

They tried it first on a chimpanzee.

The anesthetized primate was strapped on the sled with head pointing forward, blasted down the track, and brought to a 270-G stop.

The remains of the chimp were, as one officer later put it, a mess. There was no second test, and humans never tried it.

In fact, animals rode the sled much more often than men, attained much higher velocities, and were subjected to much greater G forces. Some simply vanished, disintegrated by the air blast.

The high-stress animal tests led Dr. Stapp to one of his most valuable conclusions about the nature of G forces, and their effect on the body.

One of the things the aircraft designers needed to know was how much punishment a pilot could stand before he began to sustain disabling injury. A few bruises were acceptable in a combat situation, for instance, but an injury that disabled a pilot, even for a moment, could be fatal. How far could the body be pushed?

That information could be critical in designing life support systems, ejection seats, and cockpits for the new Mach 2 aircraft now on the drawing boards.

Using first the sled in California and later the bigger, faster one in New Mexico, the Stapp group subjected animals to a variety of speeds and braking forces. At very high Gs the animal simply came apart. At lower Gs, they sustained minor bruises.

After each test, Dr. Stapp and his team pored over the autopsy results and compared them to the data collected by the monitors. As time passed and the information base grew, they massaged the information into graphs and equations. Somewhere in the abstract mathematics, Dr. Stapp felt certain, he would find clues to help him predict injuries and, then, prevent them.

In this effort, photographs of the run and impact were critical. Only in that way could the scientists correlate the graphs and equations with what was happening to the animal—or man—in the sled.

The photographs came from high-speed cameras. One camera was carried aboard the chase plane that followed the rocket sled down the track. The other was mounted on the very nose of the sled, facing backward, aimed at the occupant of the seat.

Because of the short exposure times involved, the high-speed cameras required a great deal of illumination. That was one of the advantages of doing the work at Holloman AFB in Alamogordo. The sun always shined at Alamogordo.

Well, almost always.

Now Dr. Stapp sat in *Sonic Wind Number One* and waited. The photographers loitered around the jeeps. The mechanic leaned on the sled.

Dr. Stapp squinted at the sky in front of him. Because his head was immobilized he couldn't look up. Was it his imagination, or did the sky seem a little brighter?

Were the clouds thinning?

It was getting much warmer, but no one offered Dr. Stapp anything to drink. Once, years ago, while waiting for a sled run, one of the crew members had passed around coffee and doughnuts. He offered some to Dr. Stapp.

"No, thank you," the flight surgeon replied, looking down the track. "A full stomach makes for a messy autopsy."

After that, nobody offered.

Finally, as the early animal tests had proceeded, the answer appeared, as Dr. Stapp knew it would, in the equations. There was a relationship between a killing dose of Gs and a safe one.

Specifically, it took about one fourth as much energy to injure an animal as it did to kill it. If a hog or a bear died at 200 Gs, for instance, it wouldn't sustain any injury at all up to about 50 Gs.

Dr. Stapp called that upper limit of safety the "point of beginning injury." Hogs and bears were about the same size as humans, so humans should also be able to sustain 50 Gs without permanent harm.

The point of beginning injury.

That was the limit Dr. Stapp would probe today, if only the sun would come out.

Five minutes. Just five minutes.

The jeep ran down the track again, honking.

The pools of water at the far end of the sled run were part of a new braking system designed after the mechanical system had failed.

The undercarriage of the sled was equipped with big scoops that broke through the fragile dams and hurled the water into the air, absorbing the energy and bringing the sled to a stop. By varying the size and depth of the pools between the tracks, the scientists could apply exactly the braking force they needed, at the time they needed it.

The new system brought the sled to a halt in a cloud of white fog. The photographers loved it.

A technician passed the time by rechecking the wire that ran from the blockhouse, behind the sled, to the detonators on the rockets. Dr. Stapp studied the sky before him.

Clouds. Over Alamogordo. Alamogordo!

The reporters and photographers collected legends about the sled and the early runs, and while they made good copy they often angered Dr. Stapp. As a scientist, he was offended by the untrue.

For instance, there was the story about the chimps who made repeated runs. As the legend put it, the second time a chimp was taken to the sled he "went ape." That was hogwash, of course. The animals weren't frightened of the sled at all, because they never saw it. They were anesthetized.

That was part of the value of human runs. When a human was strapped to the sled and fired down the track, he remembered the experience. It burned itself indelibly onto his brain.

Much of the necessary data could be collected by using the animals, but, as Dr. Stapp tried time and time again to explain to his superiors, the Air Force pilot wasn't a hog or a chimp. The pilot was a creature who had evolved to walk upright, to hold his spine straight, and to use his forelegs to work with tools. He was unique in the animal kingdom.

Was he also uniquely fragile?

To find out, humans would have to ride the sled.

There was a second aspect to human tests, as well. Scientifically, the human mind is an elegantly sensitive instrument. A man sees things a camera doesn't, feels things that don't register on the monitors, and can describe the experience afterward.

"That's the difference of doing it on a man and on an animal," Stapp explained to one reporter. "An animal can't tell you a lot of useful things. It can't tell you that the straps are too loose, or too tight, or rubbing the wrong place, for instance."

How much could a man tell you, after blasting down a track at close to the speed of sound and slapping into the equivalent of a brick wall?

Quite a lot, Dr. Stapp believed from the beginning.

True, the sudden stop at the end of the track lasted only a few milliseconds. But accident victims said that the human brain responds to stress by anesthetizing the emotion and stretching time.

At the moment of an accident, cracks seem to spread across the windshield in wondrous slow motion. A child's scream is endlessly prolonged, but curiously devoid of emotional impact. The graceful curve of the guard rail etches itself forever into the mind.

Those were the experiences of the people who hadn't

expected an impact, who weren't prepared for it.

What would happen if the animal in the sled was a well educated lieutenant colonel in the Air Force medical corps, if he knew exactly what he was going to encounter, and if he focused his mind? Such an animal might discover . . . what?

What did one of those equations *feel* like?

It was something a pilot, about to eject at Mach 2, desperately needed to know.

For Dr. Stapp, an officer in the United States Air Force, one thing was perfectly obvious from the very beginning. He wouldn't ask his men to do anything he wouldn't do himself.

An hour passed in the sled. Then another. The bright spot in the clouds climbed higher, and higher. His head immobile, the man in the seat watched the sky in front of him.

Were the clouds thinner?

They were. And whiter.

Suddenly the shadows sharpened and the sky turned blue.

"Let's go."

The mechanic leaped up on the sled and quickly checked the straps, tugging on the buckles. Dr. Stapp opened his mouth and the flight surgeon, on the other side of the sled, stuck a hard rubber bite block in it. That way, the pounding of his skull against his jaw wouldn't knock his teeth out.

The mechanic reached across and gave the wide chest strap one last tug, for safety, then jumped down from the sled and ran.

In the *Sonic Wind*, Dr. Stapp's heartbeat increased. There would be an increase in blood pressure, some trembling, perhaps. Sweating on the palms.

Data.

At least he didn't have a wife.

A wife probably would have screamed at him over the broken wrist, or, worse, cried. A wife wouldn't have understood that it was a simple medical matter. The wrist broke because the wind caught it, that's all. Dynamics.

What he had done made perfectly good medical sense. He knew instantly that the wrist was broken. He knew that the sooner it was set, the sooner it would heal, and the sooner it healed, the sooner he could get back to work.

He knew that the instant the impact was over, so he did the obvious thing. As soon as he got his breath back, he reached down, felt the bones, grabbed the wrist, steeled himself against the pain, and twisted.

Moments later a jeep slid to a halt beside the sled, and the test run's official doctor jumped up beside Dr. Stapp. But by that time there was nothing therapeutic left for him to do. The wrist was already set.

Dr. Stapp was mystified by the fuss. After all, it was his wrist. He was a doctor, wasn't he? He was qualified!

He was also unrepentant. When he broke the same wrist in a different place a few runs later, he set it again.

No, a wife would have had trouble understanding. So there was no wife.

"*Two minutes*," said the speaker.

Two red flares hissed behind the sled, arcing into the beautiful blue sky.

Dr. Stapp waited, staring down the tracks. Bright light flooded down from the beautiful blue sky, and the horizon shimmered with mirages.

If it was difficult to breathe, that was a physiological fact. A data point.

A jeep sped down the parallel road, toward the end of the track. That would be the flight surgeon. The ambulance driver cranked his starter.

"*One minute.*"

In the sled, Dr. Stapp fought for breath.

It wasn't fear.

Data:

The chest strap.

It was too tight. He couldn't breathe.

"Thirty seconds."

The chase plane would already be in the air.

The sun was bright, the sky was blue, but the clouds would soon close in again. How long would the sun shine?

Five minutes.

Overriding the sensation of suffocation, Dr. Stapp tried to alter his breathing, using the diaphragm more, taking in the air in shallow gulps.

"Twenty seconds."

The chase plane came in low, out of the mirage mountain range, its sleek shadow racing beneath it.

Dr. Stapp clasped and unclasped his hands. Sweating palms. Naturally. Data.

"Ten."

He would touch, this run, the mystical point of beginning injury. This time, he would feel the equations.

"Nine."

Of course I'm a bachelor, he told the reporters. In my business, what sane woman would have me?

"Eight."

The chase plane grew larger in the southern sky. Dr. Stapp's fingers found the cord that would turn on the high-speed cameras in front of him.

"Seven.

"Six."

Two hundred yards away, newsreel cameras began to whine.

"Five.

"Four."

The ambulance waited at the far end of the track, parked alongside the flight surgeon's jeep.

"*Three.*"

He could hear the chase plane. He forced himself to relax.

"*Two.*"

He pulled the camera cord hard.

"*One.*"

I can't breathe.

There was a clear pop as the igniters went, and then the seat smashed into his back.

The chase plane roared over the blockhouse, cameras whirring. Inside, the astonished pilot saw the sled pull ahead of him.

$E = mc^2$. Time is relative.

Time is motion and force.

He needed a reference. He needed numbers.

He must count.

One.

The focus left his eyes and the railings turned to fuzzy stripes. The horizon wavered.

The wind blasted against him like a pounding fist, deforming his body. Grains of sand buried themselves in his flesh.

Data.

Two.

Eyes.

Blackness closed in from the edges of his visual field.

The Gs crushed him against the seat.

The wind pounded him.

Data.

Three.

Eyes.

The world was black.

Six hundred thirty-two miles an hour. Burnout.

The Gs stopped. He seemed to float forward in the chair.

Data.

Four.

The first scoop hit the water and the rear segment of the rocket sled detached, falling behind. A millisecond later, the scoops on the forward section went through the next dam.

Shock.

Eyeballs.

The G forces tore at the delicate retinas of the eyes. The world turned yellow.

Five.

His body pulled forward against the straps. A powerful hand wrenched his intestines.

Gs.

Eyeballs.

The eyes.

The retinas flexed and rippled under the strain, and the world turned salmon pink.

The eyeballs.

They felt like they were coming out.

Eyelids closed, eyeballs straining against them, eyelids ballooning outward.

Pain. Eyes hurt. Pain. Pain.

Six.

Eyes.

Then it was over.

The cloud of spray settled, and was immediately absorbed by the dry dust. The chase plane disappeared into the distance.

But I can't breathe.

On the nose of the sled, the high-speed camera expended the last of its film and stopped. Lieutenant Colonel Stapp slumped forward against the harness, his face turning blue.

A jeep roared across the desert and came to a skidding

halt by the sled. The flight surgeon hit the ground running. In an instant he was on the sled, pulling out the bite block and tearing at the chest straps.

As the straps fell away, Dr. Stapp gasped for air.

I can breathe.

He tried to open his eyes.

I can breathe, but *I can't see.*

It was a numb fact, data, uncolored by emotion.

Salmon pink. The world was salmon pink.

Ammonia bit at his nostrils. Did they think he had passed out? He turned his face angrily away from the oxygen mask that the flight surgeon was trying to clamp over his nose.

"I'm all right!"

His hands, freed from the straps, went to his eyes. His fingers pried the lids open. He pointed his face at the sky.

Pink. Not blue. Pink. Salmon pink.

I can't see.

Data.

He felt the hands pull him from the sled, and he fought. He was all right. He was just blind, that's all.

Salmon pink!

The eyes. The eyes, of course.

The chimps would never have told him that!

Chimps and bears could never have told him that the point of beginning injury, to a human, wasn't marked by torn muscles, injured kidneys, or shattered bones.

No, the point of beginning injury occurred when the dispassionate forces of physics begin to tear at the retinas and wrench the eyeballs from the head.

He still had his eyeballs. His fingers told him that. But if the retinas were torn loose, he would never see again.

Data.

The news cameras clicked, taking pictures of the man who had sped across the surface of the earth with the speed of a .45 bullet, faster than anyone before him, the man who, just a few minutes ago, had become the fastest man on earth.

It had been a perfect run, flawless, without incident.

Except for the eyes, of course.

Eyes.

He waited for an emotion, but there was nothing.

It was data, all data.

Someone wrapped a blood-pressure cuff around his arm. He felt the metallic touch of the stethoscope on his chest.

Carefully, they laid him on a stretcher.

The sky.

Had the clouds closed in?

Or was the sky blue?

It wasn't pink. He knew it wasn't salmon pink.

Holding his eyelids open with his fingers, he lay on the stretcher and strained to peer through the salmon-colored haze, willed himself to see blue sky. But the world stayed pink.

He heard the door of the ambulance open. The stretcher lurched.

He stared upward.

Blind.

A speck swam in the salmon-pink haze.

He stared harder.

Was it a speck of blue?

Or imagination?

He willed the speck to resolve.

Yes, it was blue.

Blue.

And there was another. And another.

The clouds were gone.

He could see.

Deep in his mind, below the level of data, beneath the graphs and equations, an emotion stirred.

As they slid him in the ambulance Dr. John Paul Stapp stared upward, wide-eyed, into the sky, the bright sky, the clear sky, the beautiful, beautiful blue desert sky that he loved.

His twenty-ninth ride was Dr. Stapp's last. Shortly after he was released from the hospital the Air Force grounded him because, it was explained, he had become too valuable to risk. A few years later, they loaned him indefinitely to the Department of Transportation for research into automobile restraint systems.

Though the Air Force's decision to order him to stay off the sled would remain a point of bitterness until his retirement, it did have one salutary effect on his lifestyle. Not long after the order was published, he fell in love and was married.

He and his wife live today in Alamogordo, not far from the International Space Hall of Fame. The following is taken from a large plaque displayed prominently in the hall.

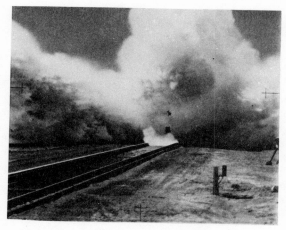

K 24–camera (500 exposures per second) head-on view of the rocket sled decelerating in the water during a 1954 run

Courtesy Dr. John Paul Stapp

John Paul Stapp
Fastest man on earth

Sled number one was ridden by Dr. John Paul Stapp in 1954 to evaluate the effects on human tissue during the extremely rapid changes in deceleration. Traveling faster than a .45 caliber bullet, reaching a peak of 632 miles per hour in 5 seconds, Dr. Stapp became known as the fastest man on earth. Deceleration changes equivalent to an open seat ejection from a cockpit at 1,800 miles per hour at 36,000 feet altitude were experienced. The space surgeon Stapp organized and founded the aeromedical facility, Edwards Air Force Base, California, and the aeromedical field laboratory, Holloman Air Force Base, New Mexico, and pioneered in research on the effects of mechanical forces on human tissue.

INDEX